"In many areas of life we become used to the status quo. Innovative ideas, while conforming to common sense, are often met with opposition because of long-established practices. *Stop the Headache* exposes the ineffective practices that have buried common-sense approaches to the debilitating pain affecting so many. It's time we open our minds to the wisdom—and health—offered here."

—*Dan Miller, life coach and author of* **Wisdom Meets Passion**

STOP THE HEADACHE

A CURE
For the Leading Cause
of Recurring Headaches and Chronic Pain

By Dr. Richard T. Seymour

Stop the Headache
©2013, Richard Seymour

Nothing written in this book should be viewed as a substitute for competent medical care. Also, you should not undertake any changes in diet or exercise patterns without first consulting your physician, especially if you are currently being treated for any medical conditions. Do not alter or stop taking prescribed medications without consulting your doctor.

For information about special discounts for bulk purchases, please contact the author at StopTheHeadache.com.

Cover design by Jeremy Seymour
Edited by Erin Casey
Copy Edited by Andrea Reynolds

Library of Congress Control Number: 2013912090
ISBN: 978-0-9832514-5-3

Covered Bridge Publishing Company
Cedarburg, Wisconsin

*To the women, elderly, and poor
around the world who are being
held captive in prisons of
pain, drugs, and medical bills.*

CONTENTS

Part III

Hope for Chronic Pain Sufferers

FOREWORD
FROM Jennifer Roach,
A FORMER CHRONIC PAIN SUFFERER

IF I TOLD YOU A CURE IS AVAILABLE FOR YOUR MIGRAINES, TENSION HEADACHES, BACK PAIN, NECK PAIN, SLEEP LOSS, CHRONIC FATIGUE, AND DEPRESSION, WOULD YOU BE INTERESTED? What if I told you this cure does not include surgery or prescription drugs? Would you be skeptical or maybe intrigued? Would it help to know that I have personally received this cure and I am 100 percent satisfied with the results?

When I was in seventh grade, I began to experience horrible migraines, severe vertigo, and chronic fatigue. Words cannot adequately describe the physical pain that consumed my daily life. Between seventh grade and twelfth grade I saw several different doctors. The best answer they could give me was that I had migraines. Their solution was to prescribe an array of migraine medicines. They were unable to provide any explanation or solution for my severe vertigo or chronic fatigue. The migraine medicines were a poor solution. After taking the medicine I would be forced to sleep for a couple hours because it made me so tired. When I woke up I would usually have a rebound headache caused by the medicine. The medicine did little more than take the edge off and temporarily mask the pain.

My symptoms progressively worsened. By eleventh grade, I relied on my mom to help me get ready for school every morning. I was too dizzy in the mornings to walk from my bedroom to the bathroom by myself, make breakfast, or drive to school. I kept a bell on my nightstand so I could get my mom's attention when I couldn't get up and needed help. I missed many days during high school because I was in such bad pain and unable to function due to the vertigo. I couldn't participate in many activities that "normal" high school students enjoyed. The chronic fatigue caused me to sleep at least fourteen hours every night and to take a three-hour nap every afternoon. I was heavily dependent on my parents for many things that I wished I could do for myself. The thought of going away to college and having a life of my own was a dream I never thought would come true.

In December 2002, during twelfth grade, my parents heard about Dr. Richard Seymour and the Chronic Pain Solution Center on the radio. They asked me if I would be willing to see another doctor. Reluctantly, I went to see Dr. Seymour in January 2003. From the moment we shook hands, I knew he was different from all the other doctors I had seen. I could tell just by his smile and kind greeting that he sincerely cared and had a great passion for helping people in pain.

After the examination, Dr. Seymour looked me in the eye and said he was confident he could not only cure my migraines, but he could also cure my severe vertigo and chronic fatigue. As he explained the cause of my pain and how he planned to take it away without surgery and without prescription drugs, my skepticism turned to hope. For the first time in over five pain-filled years, I not only had answers to where my symptoms came from, but I was offered a cure.

A couple weeks into the treatment, I woke up for the first time in over five years without pain, vertigo, and fatigue. I remember feeling like I was dreaming. I couldn't remember the last time I had physically felt that good. Tears of joy flooded my eyes as I explained to my mom

I didn't need her help getting ready. That morning was only the beginning to the life I never thought possible.

Ten years later, I am still free from migraines, vertigo, and chronic fatigue. Dr. Seymour's cure made it possible for me to go away to college and obtain both my bachelor's degree and my master's degree. I am now married to the man of my dreams, have a precious nineteen-month-old boy, and another baby boy on the way.

Because I had such great success with Dr. Seymour's treatment, I referred my grandmother to him. She suffered with migraines for sixty-four years. She also experienced hearing loss that required her to wear hearing aids. For years she went to nationally renowned headache clinics. Their solution to her migraines was to give her several prescription drugs. Immediately following treatment from Dr. Seymour, my grandmother went months without a migraine and was able to greatly cut back the amount of prescription drugs she took. She also experienced great improvement in her hearing.

If you or someone you love are living a life filled with migraines, tension headaches, back pain, neck pain, sleep loss, chronic fatigue, or depression take the time to read on and allow your skepticism to turn to hope. Allow yourself the chance to live a life free from pain; the life you never thought was possible. Don't settle for less than a cure when a cure is available.

INTRODUCTION

THROBBING, PIERCING, SEARING, MIND-NUMBING, DEBILITATING PAIN. For millions of people across the United States—and billions worldwide—chronic pain is part of everyday life. Although anyone can suffer from migraines and chronic pain, women, the elderly, and the poor are disproportionately affected. In fact, if you are a woman, you are three times more likely to suffer from chronic pain—pain that too many members of the medical community dismiss as hormone- or stress-related, or worse... "all in your head."

In the United States, it is estimated that 30 to 40 million Americans suffer from recurring migraines—and 75 percent of them are female. And migraines are only one type of chronic pain. Patients have come to me with symptoms mimicking those of Multiple Sclerosis and vertigo. Some experience hearing loss. Others are unable to get out of bed each day without the aid of numerous and expensive prescription drugs. These men and women come from different generations, different socioeconomic classes, different races... but they all share unbearable suffering in common.

You Don't Have to Live in Pain!

Do you have a loved one who experiences pain of this magnitude? Or, are you the one being held prisoner by pain? If so, my prayer is that this book brings you hope. Relief from chronic pain, migraines, and tension headaches is finally possible.

Many of my patients come to me frustrated or depressed because they spend so much of their time secluded in dark, quiet rooms in an effort to minimize their pain by hiding from light, noise, and other people. Some actually cry with relief when they realize that someone understands and believes that their pain is intense and real. When they are released from my care feeling 80 to 100 percent better without drugs, they are both elated that they no longer suffer from debilitating pain, and angry that other doctors prescribed pills, recommended expensive tests, and performed ineffective and unnecessary surgeries.

I am a dentist who specializes in chronic pain relief. Now, that may sound odd… a dentist who treats chronic pain? It's true. This book explains why well-trained dentists are exclusively able to treat many forms of chronic pain as well as migraines and tension headaches when medical physicians and pharmaceuticals cannot. That's because dentists are the only professionals trained to address issues related to the teeth and jaw. These unique areas are innervated by the trigeminal nerve system, the root cause of so many types of chronic pain and headaches.[16, 32, 35] Dentists work at the forefront of this new era of medicine that I call, **Headfirst Preventive Medicine.**

I have been successfully treating and curing patients of count-less symptoms for more than thirty-eight years. We have an A+ rating with the Better Business Bureau, and, more importantly, we have a long list of happy, healthy patients who are able to enjoy their daily lives. Throughout this book and in our videos at StopTheHeadache.com, you'll hear firsthand accounts from former chronic pain sufferers who have their lives back as a result of my treatment. These patients (most of them women) have no reservations about sharing the difference this cure and the absence of pain have made in their lives. I invite you to hear them tell their stories. Watch the interactive book trailer at **StopTheHeadache.com.** You can click on each patient's name to hear how much undiagnosed chronic pain affects people's lives.

Cure. That's a strong word, and it's one I avoided using for many years for fear of sounding hokey or like a snake-oil salesman. I substituted the phrase "long-term solution." But after so many years of successful treatments and ecstatic patients, I no longer feel cure is too strong a word.

The British Dictionary defines the term *cure* this way:

- To relieve a person of the symptoms of a disease or condition: he was cured of the disease. (She was cured, or relieved of her chronic pain).
- To eliminate (a disease or condition) with medical treatment.

The same dictionary defines *long-term* as:

- To occur over or relating to a long period of time.

Although the two terms are very similar, I feel long-term doesn't fully describe the results my patients and the patients of other dentists specializing in chronic pain experience. Cure, then, is the accurate word choice.

At this point, you may be asking if this cure will work for you. In Chapter Five, I provide a self-exam that will help answer that question. Once you perform this exam and take our online survey you will have a very good idea as to whether or not you are one of the billions who have been permitted to suffer with TNS- and TMJ-related pain. I say permitted because I believe this type of suffering is unnecessary.

A 1997 study of all medical issues treated for 692,707 members of Blue Cross Blue Shield of Massachusetts, compared TMJ and non-TMJ patients relative to healthcare costs across the board. The study revealed that the cost of overall medical inpatient treatment is double for TMJ patients. Costs for narcotics, anti-inflammatories and psychotropics for TMJ patients are triple that of non-TMJ patients.[36] Why wouldn't insurance companies want this examined and diagnosed? The article that cited this study noted that "no observation of TMJ disorders was made directly." In other words, although these TMJ patients are the greater utilizers of more costly healthcare services the medical community overlooked the obvious cause. I believe our online survey will reveal the same practice of neglecting to diagnose the real problem.

The signs of TNS and TMJoint related chronic pain are easy to diagnose. They should be obvious to every doctor, specialist, chiropractor, osteopath, and dentist. Unfortunately for you, the patient, these signs have been totally ignored for years. But if no one examines you for this problem, the cause will not be diagnosed, and you will just continue to be drugged to treat symptoms. Rather than treat the structures that cause chronic pain, doctors prescribe drugs to mask the pain—even though a proven and effective, drug- and surgery-free treatment is available.

Why Hasn't Your Doctor Mentioned This Treatment Before?

Chronic pain sufferers often ask, "If this treatment is so effective, why haven't I heard of it before?" That's a good question. In fact, it's the half-trillion dollar question. Throughout this book, I'll reveal **Newsworthy Truths**: facts that have been ignored or hidden by the medical, insurance, and pharmaceutical industries for decades. The Newsworthy Truths explain in plain, common-sense language how **abnormalities in the mouth affect the trigeminal nerve system—a complex nerve that plays a role in all five senses as well as balance—and are very often the root cause of chronic pain, migraines, and tension headaches.**[16, 32, 35] These truths will help you understand that the body is not exempt from the laws of nature and physics. You learn what causes pain in the first place and why it recurs. You will also learn that we can

---

NEWSWORTHY TRUTH

Throughout this book, I'll reveal **Newsworthy Truths**: facts that have been ignored or hidden by the medical, insurance, and pharmaceutical industries for decades. The Newsworthy Truths explain in plain, common-sense language how **abnormalities in the mouth affect the trigeminal nerve system—a complex nerve that plays a role in all five senses as well as balance—and are very often the root cause of chronic pain, migraines, and tension headaches.**

---

eliminate this life-altering pain when we apply these truths that have been common knowledge to physicians for decades.

In addition, some of the truths you will read explain why the money-makers in the medical industries work so hard to deny their patients access to drug-free relief. For example, my clinic received a letter recently denying coverage for a patient. The insurance company, Blue Cross Anthem, said the treatment is experimental—despite the fact that during the past thirty-eight years the company's claims analysts (and many others) have reviewed numerous progress reports from patients stating that they were 80 to 100 percent symptom-free without drugs following my treatment.

You'll also learn that the very people who should have chronic pain sufferers' best interests in mind are permitted (and in some cases encouraged by the administrators of their clinics) not to perform a simple exam or refer their patients to trained specialists who have the ability to offer lasting relief. To those who have suffered in pain for years, it doesn't make sense that the medical community has been permitted to ignore obvious problems and solutions for so long. It seems unimaginable that respected physicians would withhold a potential cure from their patients. If you are a chronic pain sufferer, I'm sure that even as you've read the past few paragraphs you've wondered how it is possible that your doctors haven't mentioned the trigeminal nerve system or the fact that trained dentists can offer a cure to your pain. And when you perform the self-exam and take our online survey, you will be shocked at the simplicity of diagnosing this issue. If you are like many of my patients, you will also be furious that no doctor has performed this exam on you before. You'll also understand the extreme importance of this situation and how much of your life has been stolen from you.

Truths You Should Know

If you knew how to eliminate the cause of your pain, or the suffering of someone you love, wouldn't you take steps to do so? In my years of practice, I've learned that my patients want to understand the reason for health problems affecting their lives and the lives of their family members. Knowledge gives you the power to make changes to improve your physical wellbeing. The truths that follow offer a preview of the knowledge you'll gain from this book. Each will be covered in greater detail in future chapters.

Truth #1: The Trigeminal Nerve System is the Recognized Cause of All Primary Headaches and Migraines.

Cover stories in *Newsweek* and *Time* focused extensively on the trigeminal nerve system (TNS) as the cause of migraine and all types of primary headaches. The *Time* story, "Preventing Headaches," published October 7, 2002,[1] actually referred to the TNS as the "migraine generator." The *Newsweek* cover story on migraines, published January 11, 1999, [2] noted that when an event activates the pain sensors in the trigeminal nerve system, it initiates a cycle that can keep migraines active for up to seventy-two hours. For some of my patients, the pain lasts an entire week.

6

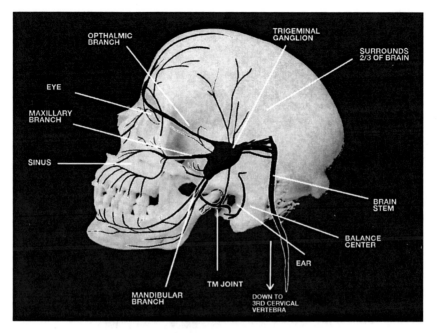

The Trigeminal Nerve System

Unfortunately, both articles discuss only one of the three major branches of the TNS, the ophthalmic branch. This branch supplies the eyes as well as a small part of the brain. The two larger branches supply the teeth, mouth muscles, jaw joints, and sinuses and the rest of the canopy surrounding the brain. If the TNS is the cause of all types of primary headaches, all three major branches of the trigeminal nerve system should be recognized as potential triggers for painful impulses throughout the brain and body.

TRUTH #2: The TNS Plays a Role in all Five Senses as well as Balance.

The three major branches of the TNS surround two-thirds of the brain like a canopy or helmet. These three branches supply the teeth, eyes, ears, sinuses, tongue, throat, neck, the masseter muscle (the strongest muscle in the body), as well as the temporalis muscle.

The temporalis muscle, which lies over the temple, is used for biting, chewing, clenching and grinding during sleep—which can explain those morning headaches. They play an integral role in the senses of sight, hearing, smell, taste, touch, and balance.

Place your fingers over your temples and clench your teeth. You'll feel this huge muscle bulge in the side of your head in the area where many of your headaches are located. If this muscle goes into spasm on both sides of the head it's like placing your head in a vice.

Truth #3: Women Are Three Times More Likely to Suffer from Headaches and Chronic Pain.

Studies show that women comprise more than 75 percent of patients suffering from migraines and chronic pain, [3, 18, 20, 36] and they are five times more likely to have a dislocated disc in their temporomandibular joint. (TMJ).[4] The literature supports the fact that women report more severe, more frequent, and longer lasting pain than men as related to temporomandibular disorders (TMD). My wife has said many times, "If this were a problem plaguing men, it would have been cured centuries ago." She's right! But instead of curing the problem, the medical community blames hormones or stress and prescribes more and more drugs to mask the symptoms.

You may ask: If hormones are not the cause of this pain—which often begins during puberty—what is the trigger? I'll provide an in-depth explanation in Chapter Three, "The Truth about the Female Epidemic of Chronic Pain and Migraines," but here's the short version. The canine teeth (also known as the cuspid or eye teeth) erupt at around age twelve or thirteen. These teeth are critical to the guidance of the mouth's closure and are responsible for relieving extreme forces on the twelve-year molars during the side-to-side movement of the lower jaw. If the canine teeth do not do their job, the twelve-year molars (which come in about the same time) are put under additional pressure. Later, between the ages of eighteen and twenty, the wisdom teeth can develop with similar

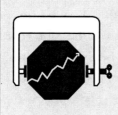

NEWSWORTHY TRUTH

The elderly don't have to continue to suffer! Many dental problems are correctable even into an individual's sixties, seventies, and eighties.

pressure/pain if the canine teeth are not in the proper position.

When you understand the simple mechanics of how this pain often starts, you can also see that a long-term cure exists for chronic pain sufferers. The mechanics makes perfect sense. What doesn't make sense is the fact that the entire medical community is permitted not to examine patients for this easy-to-diagnose condition. Instead of helping patients find a cure by referring them to a qualified dentist, they refer suffering patients to "in-house" specialists and prescribe drugs, expensive medical tests, and needless, ineffective surgeries.

TRUTH #4: The Elderly Run a Close Second to Women as the Most Abused by the Medical System.

Teeth are more than tools for chewing food. Nowhere is this more evident than with the elderly. For those in the Baby Boomer generation and older, tooth extractions were common practice. But no one has told these individuals that the extractions make them "amputees" of the skeleton of the skull or that when the teeth aren't in position, nothing prevents the jaw from over-closing. This over-closing action causes arthritis and dislocations in the TMJoints. In addition, missing and broken down teeth can influence poor head posture which often goes undiagnosed as the source of neck and back pain. Doctors and dentists neglect to explain to their patients that a misaligned bite can cause unnatural forward and lateral head posture (curvature of the spine). This posture changes weight distribution all the way down the body and alters the mechanics of every weight-bearing joint in the body.

Rather than properly diagnosing and treating, doctors tend to ignore the cause of the pain—the dislocated or arthritic TMJoints. Instead, elderly patients are given more and more drugs to cover the pain. When they can no longer deal with the constant suffering, they consent to neck surgeries, shoulder surgeries, back surgeries, and/or become so "out of it" because of the drugs that they are placed in nursing homes and long-term care facilities.

The amazing fact is that many dental problems are correctable even into an individual's sixties, seventies, and eighties. We've successfully treated patients who have suffered with migraines for forty years or more. We've treated seventy- and eighty-year-old patients with hearing and vertigo problems, and neck and back pain.

Regardless of age, people deserve to be told the truth and allowed to decide if they want to live with improved health, take fewer drugs, and experience better mental acuity and state of mind. The truth is, when people no longer live in constant pain, they often have increased longevity and undoubtedly enjoy a better quality of life.

TRUTH #5: This Problem isn't Exclusively American.

"Follow the money" is a phrase you'll read more than once in this book. In the United States, money (large sums of it) is the reason so many patients go untreated. In other countries, two things often contribute to prolonged suffering: poverty and inadequate education regarding the role of teeth as support pillars in the skull's skeleton. As a result, Third World countries use extractions as the primary treatment for tooth ailments.

When visiting with a missionary from India, I noticed she had a missing bicuspid. Curious, I asked if chronic headaches and neck pain were prevalent in India. She was shocked at my question and estimated that as much as 85 percent of the population suffered with this type of chronic pain. Even if she were only half right, that would be close to

425 million people suffering daily in India alone. I attended a course with an author from Nigeria, a country with a population of 155 million. She estimated that 70 percent of Nigerians suffer from head and neck pain. Do you understand why I say billions of people worldwide suffer from chronic pain? Because many of these countries don't keep accurate medical records on their populations, I am unable to back up these figures with scientific studies. Regardless, even if these percentages are reduced by half, a tremendous number of people suffer worldwide.

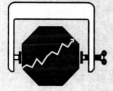 TRUTH #6: A Cure for Many Types of Chronic Pain, Migraines and Tension Headaches Has Been Available for a Very Long Time.

This cure isn't new. In Chapter One, you'll read about historical data that indicates physicians understood the connection between the teeth and headaches as many as 2,500 years ago. Many other scientifically documented discoveries about the unique nature of the TNS and TMJ have come to light in recent decades. We know, for instance, that the TNS is an extremely sensitive nerve that supplies every tooth. We know teeth play a critical role as support pillars in the skeleton of the skull and help guide the jaw to final closure. We also know the teeth are the only place in the human body where the skeleton penetrates the skin's surface. These truths allow well-trained dentists to offer a perma-

---

NEWSWORTHY TRUTH

The teeth are the only place in the human body where the skeleton penetrates the skin. This allows trained dentists to offer a permanent cure for the hellish pain of recurring headaches, migraines, neck pain, and any number of other symptoms *without surgery.*

---

nent cure for the hellish pain of recurring headaches, migraines, neck pain, and a number of other symptoms without surgery.

I'll offer much greater detail and proof to support these truths in the coming chapters, but I want you to understand now that there is an effective cure for many types of chronic pain, migraines, fibromyalgia, and tension headaches. Until now, you probably haven't even heard many of these truths nor been examined to see if the TNS could be the cause of your suffering because doctors, insurance companies and dentists are permitted to ignore obvious signs and undisputable facts.

TRUTH #7: "TMJ" is a Convenient Catchall Term, but the Real Problem is Much More Extensive.

TMJ is a catchall term that only partially describes the problems this book addresses. Don't stop reading here just because we are talking about the TMJoints (temporomandibular jaw joints located in front of the ear) and you think you've been treated for this already. This disorder is much bigger than the TMJoints; it involves the entire TNS. Part of the very sensitive trigeminal nerve runs through the TMJoints. When you consider the magnitude of this nerve's reach, it is easy to see that the chronic pain isn't simply about jaw pain and headaches. The entire TNS is the major culprit causing all sorts of recurring, chronic pain. As such, this problem—your pain—is too complex to be treated by a general dentist who dabbles in TMJ treatment.

TRUTH #8: The Medical System Frequently Prevents Diagnoses and Treatment and Keeps Patients in Pain.

Have you ever felt that doctors or the medical insurance systems contribute to prolonged pain? The truth is that clinic and hospital administrators, as well as medical insurance companies, work very hard to keep patients (a.k.a. money) "in-house." Add to that the stranglehold pharmaceutical companies have on much of the medical industry in

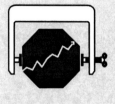

NEWSWORTHY TRUTH

Very few people will ever be diagnosed or treated for TNS- or TMJ-related pain unless doctors are forced to examine patients for these conditions and refer patients out of their in-house, self-contained clinics, hospitals, and insurance networks.

the United States, and it's no wonder millions of people have suffered with chronic pain for decades. It begins innocently, like a mild merry-go-round circling from one doctor to the next. Then the merry-go-round becomes a whirlpool of doctors and administrators dictating protocol for referrals within the system, pharmaceutical companies encouraging the sale of stronger and more expensive drugs (which contribute to doctors' or clinics' profits), and insurance companies requiring patients to stay "in-network." Sufferers are referred from specialist to specialist—none of whom offer a cure.

The following statement will be repeated throughout this book to make clear what needs to happen if this suffering is ever going to end: **Very few people will ever be diagnosed or treated for TNS- or TMJ-related pain unless doctors are forced to *examine* patients for these conditions *and refer* patients out of their in-house, self-contained clinics, hospitals, and insurance networks.** Until doctors are required to examine patients for this condition, millions of people in the United States and billions of people worldwide will continue to suffer needlessly. Until things change, hundreds of billions of dollars per year will keep rolling into the coffers of the pharmaceutical and medical industries.

Families of chronic pain sufferers have been paying the insurance premiums and footing the bill for doctor visits, drugs, and ineffective treatments for decades—largely because the true cause is never addressed. The medical and dental industries have been given a pass; they don't have to examine patients for this condition. Meanwhile, more and larger hospitals are being built and pharmaceutical companies profit primarily on the backs of women and elderly people suffering with recurring pain.

At the Chronic Pain Solution Center we address and eliminate the cause of chronic pain, migraines, and tension headaches. Rather than building a larger facility, we actually release cured patients from our care, a feat many medical practices seem incapable of performing. Our business grows because happy, healthy former patients refer new patients to us.

Most of these truths have existed for decades and are indisputable. Ignoring the truth does not change it or make it go away. Ignoring crooked or missing teeth and dislocated joints is a mistake. These issues won't resolve without proper treatment. Covering up pain with drugs or unrelated surgeries is profitable for the medical, pharmaceutical, and insurance industries, but that practice will not cure chronic pain sufferers. **In fact, masking the cause allows the collateral damage due to poor posture to worsen over decades, leading to more surgeries on weight-bearing joints such as the neck, back, hips, and knees.**

It's Time to Free the Multitudes from a Prison of Pain!

My desire with this book is to free the multitudes from pain. To do that, you and I together are going to have to force the medical, insurance, and pharmaceutical industries to acknowledge that a very real, easily detectable, and treatable condition causes billions of people to suffer daily. This book is all about truths concerning chronic pain and will empower you with knowledge. I implore you to take that knowledge and confront your physician and insurance carriers. Ask why treatment issues surrounding the trigeminal nerve system, the mouth, and the

TMJoints and are only covered by insurance in twenty-two states. (Even in those states, the insurance coverage is very poor, unlike the coverage for other joints that are less complicated and less vital to life.) When we unite and demand that the medical industry recognize the cause of so much suffering, we can force insurance companies, doctors, and medical establishments to offer a real cure.

It won't be easy to change the way this highly profitable system operates. Let me share a story that reveals how these outdated opinions affect real human lives. Ten years ago, a high school sophomore girl was being treated for migraines by a panel of specialists at a prominent hospital in Milwaukee, WI. Unable to relieve her severe headaches except with very strong medication, they recommended she drop out of high school for a trimester. She did, with no success. Her mother, who I had treated ten years earlier for migraines, finally brought her to my practice at the Chronic Pain Solution Center. The sad reality is that the girl's mother didn't bring her in earlier because she was in the midst of a divorce, and while insurance would cover the hospital, doctors, and drugs, it would not cover treatment of a dislocated joint situated just two millimeters from the brain. Within two weeks of beginning treatment at my clinic, 90 percent of her migraines were eliminated without drugs. We kept her pain-free for two and a half months without drugs; then we did a bite analysis to determine how to make the results permanent.

During this time the hospital had the girl come back to meet with the panel of doctors who had worked with her earlier. But the meeting actually wasn't about the girl. The doctors repeatedly asked the mother, "What did he do?" She described the treatment and told them how it had

---

*"Then you will know the truth
and the truth will set you free."*
—John 8:32 (NIV)

---

eliminated her own migraines years before as well. Guess how many requests for meeting or lectures I received from this panel of doctors? Zero! Guess how many children—our most cherished commodity—they've referred to me in the past ten years for treatment of migraines or neck pain? Zero! Instead, they keep their patients "in-house" and dependent on prescription drugs for some semblance of relief. How many young lives and families were ruined by pain, prescriptions, surgeries, depression, and suicides from all the drugs during those ten years? Where does this practice of pain for profit end?

How sad is it that so many people suffer daily—for decades—while those in the medical, insurance, and pharmaceutical companies profit? I realize that many members of the medical community will not like this book because of the truths revealed within. That's fine with me. This book is not intended to honor the "professionals" who have abused their calling to treat and heal the sick and suffering. This book IS intended to help the billions of chronic pain sufferers and their families. While I have been eliminating horrific symptoms for thirty-eight years, the medical community as a whole has been allowed to ignore the leading cause of chronic pain, migraines, and tension headaches. Through the years I've tried educating doctors and administrators, but now I realize it is not a matter of education. Many, if not most, professionals in this industry are aware of and understand the problem. But because the current "accepted" treatments, tests, medicines, and surgeries offered bring in hundreds of billions of dollars annually they ignore the real cure and hold millions of Americans in prisons of pain.

"Loyalty to a petrified opinion
never broke a chain
or freed a human soul."
—Mark Twain

We need to break the chains and free the multitudes! And the battle begins by sharing the truth about chronic pain. We must stand up to the system and yell, "This has to stop!" Until that happens, needless pain will continue. You have a wonderful opportunity to leave your footprints on eternity by expressing your anger and love—anger for the lives that have been stolen, and love for future generations. Because large parts of this problem are hereditary, future generations of daughters and grand-daughters will spend their lives in the same prison of pain, drugs, and financial struggles resulting from endless medical bills for treatments that only mask the problem without addressing the cause. Let's stand up and work together to force the medical community and insurance companies to examine and cover the jaw, TMJoints, and necessary dental work to stop this pain. Women are going to have to start a new "suffer-age movement" demanding their medical rights. Likewise, the elderly and poor—and those who love and care for them—must make their voices heard. The practice of pain for profit will not stop until the healthcare industry is forced to consider Headfirst Preventive Medicine before prescribing expensive and dangerous drugs and surgeries.

Existing traditional treatments reveal a biased loyalty to petrified opinions. All of us—patients, doctors, and dentists, as well as adminis-trators and insurance carriers—must abandon these misguided opinions. Until that happens, people of all ages will continue to suffer needlessly.

 ## STOP THE SUFFERING!
Help Spread the Message of This Book
Before the Medical Giants Find a Way to Stop It!

If you understand the simple mechanics and truths about teeth, the TNS and how it causes chronic pain, migraines, and tension headaches, it's easy to see how much life is stolen from suffering patients and their families. When you add up the hundreds of billions of dollars reaped each year by the rulers of the pain industry (a.k.a. healthcare system), it is clear how much is at stake for these companies. The Goliaths who profit from chronic pain don't want patients to know about this cure. We could actually have a world-changing branch of medicine that heals, stops pain, and prevents it from recurring without drugs or surgeries. We could form a preventive medical/dental specialty that would work to prevent these painful symptoms from ever recurring. You'd think that those who claim to be healers would want this information to be available to the masses… but sadly, money talks. That's why I need your help in getting the message of this book out to those who need relief—before the giants find a way to stop it.

My desire is to put an end to the practice of keeping suffering people and their families imprisoned in prisons of pain, drugs, and endless medical bills.

This problem is so big that the word epidemic doesn't cover it. It really is a worldwide pandemic. I rarely go anywhere or talk to anyone who doesn't have the problem themselves or know someone who does. I need your help to stop the suffering. Everyone reading this book has the ability to help us spread this information around the world. I know in my heart that when we create a firestorm by sharing these truths, we can initiate real change in the medical system and, ultimately, help billions of people worldwide find real relief from chronic suffering.

At the end of this book you'll learn more about how you can be part of a revolution that frees people from the antiquated rules of a broken healthcare system. In the meantime, I encourage you to:

- Take the self-exam and encourage others you know to do the same.

- Take the online survey. We want to know if you've ever been properly examined for TMJ- and TNS-related pain.

- Share facts from this book with your friends, family members, co-workers, political leaders, doctors, and dentists.

- Recommend *Stop the Headache* to the people in your life who suffer from chronic pain, migraines, and tension headaches.

- Use social media sites like Facebook and Twitter to help us spread the word.

- Contact us at **help@stoptheheadache.com** so we can coordinate the effort to challenge the practice of pain for profit within the medical profession, the medical insurance industry, the drug companies, the dental profession, and Congress.

- "Like" us on Facebook at Facebook.com/StopTheHeadache to stay current on new research and policies.

- Follow us on Twitter at twitter.com/stoptheheadache to stay up to date on new research and policies.

- Tweet quotes from this book that resonate with you. Use the hashtag #StopTheHeadache.

- Watch and share the interactive book trailer at StopTheHeadache.com.

Let's start a firestorm across the Internet! Massive groups of people and rapid information dissemination each are powerful on their own, but combined they are unstoppable. Help us spread the truths in this book and make this message unstoppable. There is a cure for many types of chronic pain, migraines, and tension headaches. Let the truth be heard and let the healing begin!

PART I

TRUTHS YOU SHOULD KNOW
About
Chronic Pain, Migraines, and Tension Headaches

News Flash:
It Is *Not* all in Your Head!

"I had been living in a virtual vortex of pain for many years and had begun to believe I would never live to see a pain-free day or night so long as I resided on planet earth. I never considered suicide, but I recall many days asking God to please heal me or take me home.

"I applied ice packs on my neck nightly and took as many pain medications as I could get my hands on. I also consumed entirely too much alcohol and am grateful I did not become an alcoholic. Many thousands of dollars were spent on massage therapists, physicians, Rolfers, acupuncturists, electric shock treatments, a TENS [Transcutaneous Electrical Nerve Stimulation] unit at home, and many chiropractors. I was taken to the hospital by ambulance at least once a year for severe back spasms and kept on morphine injections for seven to ten days until the spasms subsided. I never traveled without muscle relaxers and pain meds.

"One chiropractor eventually told me it was all in my head. He was right, but not in the way he meant. I was so offended and hurt to be labeled a hypochondriac. I was already dealing with enough pain without having the guilt of a doctor telling me I was faking it."

—Nancy Lynn, former chronic pain sufferer

IF YOU ARE A CHRONIC PAIN OR MIGRAINE SUFFERER, I WANT YOU TO KNOW I DO NOT BELIEVE YOU ARE A HYPOCHONDRIAC. The pain you feel is not "all in your head." If that's how physicians or even your exasperated family members and friends have made you feel, you are not alone. If you've been to doctor after doctor, specialist after specialist, endured tests and surgeries, and have been prescribed a series of pills that make you feel foggy, sleepy but offer little relief, you are not alone.

After years of suffering with chronic pain, many people begin to believe the white-coat doctors who say their misery is psychosomatic. I believe that the doctors who tell their patients that the pain is all in their heads, or that they're depressed, or that they can't cope with the stress of life would become moody and irritable as well if they had to deal with severe pain every day!

When suffering individuals enter that dark room (dungeon) to deal with this horrific pain, they feel they are alone in the battle. That is the definition of hell in anyone's language. Nancy Lynn was suffering in that kind of hell when she first came to my office more than twenty years ago. Today, happy and healthy at seventy years young, she remains enthusiastic about the immediate relief that is available for chronic pain sufferers. In her words:

"It was heaven! Unbelievable! I had forgotten how it felt to be pain-free. After so many years of treatment, bills, drugs, and alcohol, I was being lifted out of this endless pit of pain. I actually wanted to live again. My high energy level returned. It is so very sad that so many suffer so much and so needlessly. I am so grateful to God I found a doctor who is so knowledgeable about TMJ and that we could afford the treatments because our insurance would not touch it. When I see people with my same problem or with migraines, I try to tell them about the cure, but they know nothing about the TMJ and the damage it can do to the entire body. This treatment is the best kept secret in the medical, pharmaceutical, and sadly, even in the dentistry world. That is criminal. My entire journey

Common Symptoms of Chronic Pain Related to the Trigeminal Nerve System

- Constant recurring severe headaches (tension, cluster, sinus, stress, and/or morning headaches)
- Migraines
- Stabbing eye pain and visual symptoms
- Ear pain, hearing loss, tinnitus (ringing/noise in the ear)
- Sinus problems
- Neck and shoulder pain
- Back pain
- Facial pain or burning (trigeminal neuralgia)
- Temporomandibular Joint pain (jaw pain)
- Fibromyalgia
- Snoring
- Poor sleep and sleep apnea
- Vertigo or dizziness

Several other chronic conditions are being traced back to the TNS. For example, we know of two patients who were told they had Multiple Sclerosis (MS). After removing stress on the TNS via the TMJoints the MS symptoms disappeared. Additionally, doctors are seeing very encouraging results for patients with Parkinson's and Tourette's by relieving pressure on the TNS branch in back of the TMJoints.[37]

In addition to all the symptoms listed above, when chronic pain takes over a patient's life, chronic fatigue and depression are generally constant companions.

When medicine and dentistry come to grips with the reality that all the vital senses and sections of the brain and brainstem that the TNS relays impulses to and from are connected, we should not be surprised to see a solution for dementia and Alzheimer's in the future. My desire is to start a research foundation that studies the TNS to provide treatment and cures for these conditions so people will not be forced to take drugs that only dull the symptoms.

through this abyss of pain is nothing short of a miracle to me, and I will be ever grateful for Dr. Seymour and his mission to change the problem of pain as so many know it."

This "problem of pain" is real, and I am on a two-fold mission to end it. The first part of that mission is to help you find the cure for your pain without drugs or surgeries. The second part of that mission is to force doctors, dentists, insurance executives, and administrators to acknowledge and treat the cause of this pain and suffering. In both cases, understanding the cause of chronic pain is the first step to healing.

IT'S A MATTER OF ENGINEERING

The laws of physics, mechanics and gravity are true anywhere in the world, even in the human body. Ask the elderly about gravity and they'll give you an earful. But few of them realize how the law of gravity can cause changes in posture—and that those changes often result in pain. Postural changes—for example, forward head positioning and curvature of the spine—and the pain they cause are one of countless symptoms that can be brought on by structural engineering problems in the body. More specifically, it's the engineering of mouth, teeth, and, in the skeleton and nervous system of the head, TMJoints and muscles of mastication where many issues start. The primary reason for the pain is that these critical areas are all controlled by the TNS.

Your mouth plays an essential role in your well-being. It gives you the ability to eat, drink, talk, sing, and kiss. While those actions are vital, your mouth, jaw, and teeth are even more important to your health. If you have ever had a tooth pulled, particularly a molar, or if your teeth are sensitive, broken, damaged, or misaligned, your mouth can also be the source of excruciating pain. That's because your teeth serve as support pillars for your jaw.

Consider the structural support and accuracy of engineering necessary to keep a skyscraper standing. The human body, like a skyscraper, is subject to the laws of structural engineering and gravity. If you remove a support beam from a skyscraper, the building's other support beams would be forced to take on additional weight. Over time, those over-loaded pillars would bend or crack under the strain. Eventually, if not repaired, those beams would collapse and cause enormous amounts of collateral damage.

In the same way, missing molars or a misaligned bite put undue stress and pressure on the Temporomandibular Joints (TMJ). This stress irritates the trigeminal nerve system (TNS) which, in turn, leads to migraines and a range of chronic pain symptoms including neck and shoulder pain, back aches, eye pain, vertigo, sleep apnea, fibromyalgia, hearing loss, and more.

If that list of varied symptoms sounds unlikely, consider this: The TNS is the largest of the twelve cranial nerves. Like a canopy, it surrounds two-thirds of the brain. I'll give you more specifics about the TNS later, but for now you need to know that this amazing nerve system supplies and plays a role in the function of the eyes, ears, sinuses, throat, tongue, chewing muscles, both jaw joints, all of the teeth, and the upper and lower jaw bones down to the third cervical vertebra of the neck. It is unique in that it is both a motor nerve and the chief sensory nerve of the head and face.

NEWSWORTHY TRUTH

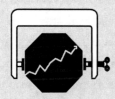

The **Trigeminal Nerve System** (TNS) surrounds two-thirds of the brain and is the largest of the twelve cranial nerves. It supplies and plays a role in the function of the eyes, ears, sinuses, throat, tongue, chewing muscles, both jaw joints, all of the teeth, and the upper and lower jaw bones down to the third cervical vertebra of the neck. It is unique in that it is both a **motor nerve** and the **chief sensory nerve** of the head and face.

To understand just one way the TNS operates and can cause pain, fan your fingers over your temples and clench your teeth. The muscle you feel bulging under your fingers is the temporalis muscle, which works in conjunction with the masseter muscle, the strongest muscle in the body. Both of these powerful muscles, along with other muscles used for chewing and clenching, are controlled by the TNS. It's noteworthy that the temporalis muscle lies directly over the temple area where many people experience migraine headaches. When the TNS is irritated it can send the temporalis muscle into spasm causing headaches so severe that lights and sounds are unbearable. When we are able to stop many of the irritations to the TNS we are often able to end pain without drugs.

THE INESCAPABLE LAW OF GRAVITY

Back to the engineering of the body… A stone in your shoe causes you to limp. Imagine the issues that limp would cause if the stone remained in your shoe for years. Eventually you would experience knee pain, hip pain and lower back pain. What do you think might happen if your TMJoints are dislocated, or your teeth are crooked, or sensitive to pressure, hot or cold, or if you are missing teeth? Like an irritating stone, these issues precipitate pain avoidance. You unconsciously chew on one side and avoid the other. If this goes on for an extended period of time you will likely tip your head forward and off to one side.[5, 6, 7] You are now a skyscraper with a penthouse apartment out over the front and side of the building, rather than perfectly aligned on top. This head posture combines with another inescapable law to work against you: the law of gravity.

If you have a forward or lateral head posture—ask a friend or relative if you do—your neck and back are battling gravity most of the day. If you have a deep overbite (see the self-exam) and a Class Two malocclusion; retruded lower jaw and small chin, it is unlikely that your head will be directly over the midline of your body, right to left and front to back. Poor head posture like this has more to do with developing a dowager's hump in your upper spine more than osteoporosis! That's because at eleven to

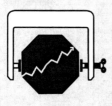

NEWSWORTHY TRUTH

Poor head posture has more to do with developing curvature of the spine and a dowager's hump than osteoporosis. That's because the weight of the head doubles for each inch it is forward or off to one side.

sixteen pounds, your head weighs as much as a bowling ball. If it's off midline at the top of the human skyscraper, its weight is doubled for every inch it is forward or off to a side.[5, 8] Now add the weight of your neck and rounded shoulders that usually follow as the poor posture works its way down your body. The amount of weight straining your lower back, hips, and knees is enormous. If your head is forward and your eyes aren't focused on the horizon, and your balance is negatively affected, it can lead to vertigo, which is the most crippling symptom of all—you can't drive, you can't work, you can't care for your kids.

Physics, Simple Mechanics & Your Body

The laws of physics have governed the way things function since the beginning of time. The same common-sense laws that apply to simple machines also apply to the mouth and the rest of the human body. Take a look at these illustrations to better understand how the mechanics of your mouth work.

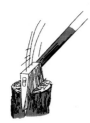

Axe: The axe or cusp tips (wedges) split food. But if the two teeth colliding don't line up properly, the opposing teeth become sensitive at the point of impact. In worse case scenarios, the cusp tips of one tooth fractures or splits the opposing molar.

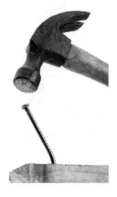

Hammer: What happens when you strike a nail off-center with a hammer? A glancing strike bends the nail. In the mouth, when a crooked lower tooth glances off the fixed upper tooth the entire lower jaw, all the chewing muscles and both joints are displaced out of their triplane comfort zone at the last second of impact, hundreds of times per day. That number increases significantly if you grind your teeth at night during sleep.

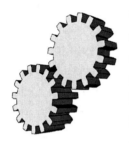

Gears: Most machines don't run if a cog is missing or the gears are crooked. The cusp tips of the teeth of the lower jaw are like cogs or gear teeth designed to line up with the cusp tip of the lower arch directly. The body won't function at its best when the lower jaw glances off teeth that don't line up.

If the condyle of the lower jaw is over-closing in the joints because teeth are missing and you don't have the proper vertical support pillars in the skeleton of the skull to prevent this from damaging the joints, the gears of your mouth are not working with optimal precision.

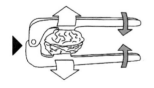

Punch Press: I think you'll agree the opposing arches of teeth are like a punch press, poking holes in food. If the moveable lower arch of teeth doesn't mesh with the upper fixed arch of teeth, there will be a glancing (scraping) motion that occurs. How long do you think the opposing tables of a punch press will last if the projections don't line up exactly? The mouth is no different. Teeth will become sensitive, feeling like they need a root canal. It will destroy bone around the teeth that don't line up and cause gum disease, or the tooth will fracture. Just as the punch press glances off in the last second of impact, what do you think happens inside both TMJoints? Both will be displaced.

Nutcracker: Forces in a nutcracker become significantly greater as they get closer to the joint between the two lever arms. While you can't crack a nut at the end of the handle, near the joint you need to apply very little pressure to crack the nut because the forces there are so much greater. Similarly, the forces in the back of the mouth—in the area of the molars—are much greater than at the front of the mouth. Combine the simple mechanics of leverage with the strongest muscle in the body, the masseter muscle, which is just outside the molar areas, and the pressure will equate to hundreds of pounds per square inch. The Guinness World Record of these forces is 965 pounds per square inch! The normal range is around 140 pounds per square inch. For those who suffer from migraines and recurring headaches, the pressure is closer to 250 to 300 pounds per square inch. That's more than many people weigh!

A BALANCED BITE IS CRITICAL TO YOUR HEALTH

The TMJoints and molars take on the stress of a weight-bearing joint. No wonder teeth are covered with the hardest structure in the human body. The pressure they withstand is enormous.

Ill-fitting bites are a major contributor to fractured teeth, root canals, and tooth loss due to gum disease (destruction of the bone) which surrounds the teeth that are traumatically colliding all day long. Flossing is important in the prevention of gum disease. One important truth you must understand regarding the cure for chronic pain is that the teeth are the only place in the human body where the skeleton comes through the skin. A well-trained dentist using modern technology including bite computers can alter or restore the skeleton to make these simple machines (your teeth, upper and lower jaw) work in perfect balance the way they are supposed to.

Since 1992, we have used a high-tech bite computer, the TekScan III, in our clinic to find areas of undue stress in the mouth. In my opinion, every dentist, periodontist, endodontist, orthodontist, and oral surgeon should have one of these computers because they provide the information needed for the prevention of premature tooth loss, sensitivity, gum disease, and decades of chronic pain. Sadly, I have yet to have a new patient show up in our office during the past twenty years and say, "Oh, my dentist has one of those computers." Please note: I am not a vendor or an affiliate for TekScan®. I do not get any royalties or kickbacks from them; I just know the miracles this product has produced in my practice. For example, I am very proud to say that no patient in my practice with a reasonable complement of teeth has ever ended up with dentures, except for one who was the victim of sixteen surgeries on her TMJoints by other practitioners.

With this computer, we can balance mouths down to thousands of a millimeter, and we can time the guidance systems to reduce the torque on teeth to such an extent that we can prevent bone loss, gum disease, and fractures that lead to root canals, tooth loss, bridges, partials and eventually dentures.

THE SIDE EFFECTS OF PAIN

Just as the TNS can cause pain in many areas of the body, pain itself can have far-reaching consequences. For example, nonstop pain drains a person's energy to the point that he or she is unable to participate in everyday activities. Mood swings, a side effect from drugs and from simply never feeling good, almost always have a negative effect on spousal relationships and friendships. Absenteeism due to recurring pain can lead to job loss and financial issues. And let's not forget the financial prison of never-ending medical bills for drugs and procedures that don't address the cause. Take a look at a few of the ways chronic pain has a negative impact on a person's quality of life.

Migraine Facts[3]

36 million people—about 18 percent of American women and 6 percent of American men—suffer from migraines. This equates to 27 million women who suffer from migraines.

Migraines rank in the top 20 of the world's most disabling medical illnesses.

In nearly one in four U.S. households someone suffers with migraines. This truth equates to entire families being held prisoners to the pain financially because of repeated doctor's appointments, emergency room visits, and prescription costs.

More than 90 percent of sufferers are unable to work or function normally during their migraine attacks.

While most sufferers experience attacks once or twice a month, about 14 million people experience headaches on a near-daily basis.

American employers lose more than $13 billion each year as a result of 113 million lost work days.

Poor and Interrupted Sleep

This pain is often bad enough that it keeps patients from sleeping or wakes them in agony.

Chronic Fatigue

Many of these patients never reach the critical REM (rapid eye movement) state of sleep, so they are never, or rarely, fully rested. Even if they are able to get a full night's sleep, ongoing pain during the day robs them of their energy. Simply going through the motions of daily activities leaves them exhausted because so much of their energy is consumed with combating pain.

Feelings of Depression or Despondency

Lack of sleep can also lead to feelings of depression. *Will I ever feel good again?* is a question many chronic pain sufferers ask daily. With no relief in sight, they withdraw from loved ones, hiding alone in dark rooms in an attempt to escape the pain. Of course, the medical profession's response is to prescribe antidepressants and sleep medications that make the patient more fatigued.

Complications from Medications

Prescription medications can be beneficial if they're prescribed for the right reason. Masking symptoms while not addressing the cause of the pain only exacerbates the problem. In addition to the expense, drugs can cloud the patient's life and create long-term side effects, systemic complications, and needless abdominal surgeries years later.

Job Loss

Patients with temporomandibular disorders (TMD) have high levels of unemployment and decreased work effectiveness. A large, population-based, cross-sectional study showed that TMD chronic pain had an impact and burden similar to that of back pain, severe headaches, and chest and abdominal pain.

Financial Burdens

Sixty-two percent of all personal bankruptcies filed in the United States in 2007 were caused by medical problems according to a study by Harvard researchers cited in *The American Journal of Medicine* (Volume 122, Issue 8). The cost of medical bills, prescriptions, and lost time at work all add up to a huge burden on the patient and his or her family. And while health insurance may help in some cases, the same study found that 78 percent of those who had filed for bankruptcy had medical insurance—at least at the start of their illness. Let's not forget the financial burden of disability on governments.

Craniomandibular Pain Syndrome

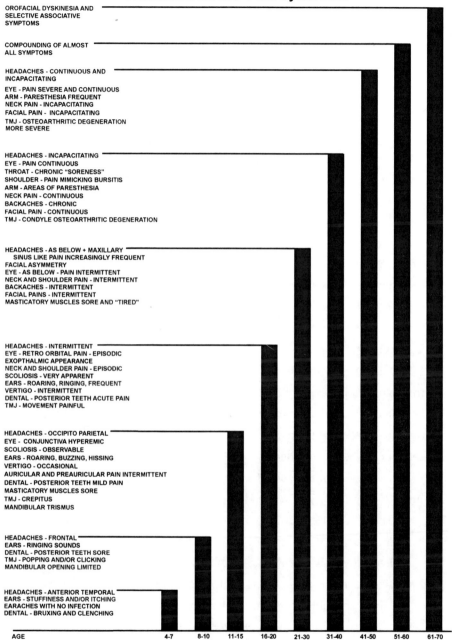

OROFACIAL DYSKINESIA AND
SELECTIVE ASSOCIATIVE
SYMPTOMS

COMPOUNDING OF ALMOST
ALL SYMPTOMS

HEADACHES - CONTINUOUS AND
INCAPACITATING
EYE - PAIN SEVERE AND CONTINUOUS
ARM - PARESTHESIA FREQUENT
NECK PAIN - INCAPACITATING
FACIAL PAIN - INCAPACITATING
TMJ - OSTEOARTHRITIC DEGENERATION
MORE SEVERE

HEADACHES - INCAPACITATING
EYE - PAIN CONTINUOUS
THROAT - CHRONIC "SORENESS"
SHOULDER - PAIN MIMICKING BURSITIS
ARM - AREAS OF PARESTHESIA
NECK PAIN - CONTINUOUS
BACKACHES - CHRONIC
FACIAL PAIN - CONTINUOUS
TMJ - CONDYLE OSTEOARTHRITIC DEGENERATION

HEADACHES - AS BELOW + MAXILLARY
SINUS LIKE PAIN INCREASINGLY FREQUENT
FACIAL ASYMMETRY
EYE - AS BELOW - PAIN INTERMITTENT
NECK AND SHOULDER PAIN - INTERMITTENT
BACKACHES - INTERMITTENT
FACIAL PAINS - INTERMITTENT
MASTICATORY MUSCLES SORE AND "TIRED"

HEADACHES - INTERMITTENT
EYE - RETRO ORBITAL PAIN - EPISODIC
EXOPTHALMIC APPEARANCE
NECK AND SHOULDER PAIN - EPISODIC
SCOLIOSIS - VERY APPARENT
EARS - ROARING, RINGING, FREQUENT
VERTIGO - INTERMITTENT
DENTAL - POSTERIOR TEETH ACUTE PAIN
TMJ - MOVEMENT PAINFUL

HEADACHES - OCCIPITO PARIETAL
EYE - CONJUNCTIVA HYPEREMIC
SCOLIOSIS - OBSERVABLE
EARS - ROARING, BUZZING, HISSING
VERTIGO - OCCASIONAL
AURICULAR AND PREAURICULAR PAIN INTERMITTENT
DENTAL - POSTERIOR TEETH MILD PAIN
MASTICATORY MUSCLES SORE
TMJ - CREPITUS
MANDIBULAR TRISMUS

HEADACHES - FRONTAL
EARS - RINGING SOUNDS
DENTAL - POSTERIOR TEETH SORE
TMJ - POPPING AND/OR CLICKING
MANDIBULAR OPENING LIMITED

HEADACHES - ANTERIOR TEMPORAL
EARS - STUFFINESS AND/OR ITCHING
EARACHES WITH NO INFECTION
DENTAL - BRUXING AND CLENCHING

AGE   4-7   8-10   11-15   16-20   21-30   31-40   41-50   51-60   61-70

* An evolutionary, progressive and cumulative clinical index pattern correlated from symptoms documented in craniomandibular pain patients by Dr. Lawrence
A. Funt (Bethesda, Maryland) and Dr. Brendan C. Stack (Falls Church, Virginia) — Directors of the National Capital Center for Craniofacial Pain.

Contributing Authors: "The Clinical Management of Head, Neck and Jaw Dysfunction" as published by the W. B. Saunders Company, December 1977.

Damaged Relationships and Broken Marriages

Jill B. is a former chronic pain sufferer who knows firsthand how life consuming this *TNS-related* pain can be. "For fourteen years my chronic headaches, dizziness, neck, and facial pain dominated my life," she says. "I saw many specialists, surgeons, and psychiatrists. They hospitalized me for months at a time for depression and fatigue, and I endured electric shock therapy numerous times. Medical bills of $250,000 forced us into bankruptcy, and I was still in pain. Then I found the Chronic Pain Solution Center. The cause of the pain was relieved, my depression decreased, my energy improved, and I got my life back."

Worse yet, the pain and difficulties associated with TNS and TMJoints are progressive. Take a look at the chart on page 35 to see how the number and severity of symptoms increases with age if the problem goes undiagnosed and/or untreated.

CHRONIC PAIN: TRUTHS THROUGH THE AGES

Lest you think I'm proposing a discovery or medical break-through — let me explain the truth about how long some of this information has been available: information that could have helped relieve you or your loved ones from chronic pain years ago. Although I'm primarily referencing headaches here, you've already seen a long list of symptoms that are related directly or referred indirectly via the TNS and the structures it supplies as well as head posture.

These historic studies will undoubtedly leave you asking: Why have these truths been ignored for centuries?

Let's start 2,500 years ago with Hippocrates, the Father of Modern Medicine and author of the Hippocratic Oath that all physicians take when they graduate from medical school. In his writings twenty-five centuries ago, Hippocrates observed a very important fact. He noted that patients whose teeth were crooked or crowded are "molested by headaches and otorrhea (discharge from the external ear)."[7, 10] All those

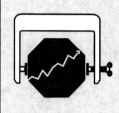

NEWSWORTHY TRUTH

Half a century ago treatment by altering the occlusion and repositioning of the lower jaw was successful in over 75 percent of all cases.

centuries ago, Hippocrates understood that people with crooked or misaligned teeth were more prone to recurring headaches and ear problems.

Dr. Harry Campbell, a physician from the early 1900s, who I believe should get the Nobel Prize for medicine posthumously, figured out the source of chronic headaches and referred pain even before the medical world had any real understanding of the TNS. Back as far as 1894 in his text titled "Headache and Other Morbid Cephalic (relating to the head) Sensations,"[8] Campbell references writings from the 1750s that made the connection between teeth and head pain. The quote I must point out from Campbell's book is this: "That abnormal states of the teeth may cause faceache and neuralgic pains in other parts of the head is a fact familiar to all, and has been, from the earliest days of medicine." Why, if this fact were "familiar to all" in 1894, is it not known today? He quotes another physician, Lauder Brunton, who "emphasized the important part played by dental irritation in the causation of headache. 'In all cases of headache, the first thing I do is examine the teeth.'"

Campbell also noted that pain with dental origins often presents itself, or is referred, as a different symptom entirely. In "Disorders of the Teeth," Campbell wrote, "It is not, however, so generally known that head-pain, having no apparent connection with the teeth, may have a dental origin, the pain being felt, not at this actual source of the irritation, but at some distance from it, so that the patient, as Lauder Brunton puts it, 'gets the toothache in another part of the head.'" Campbell also

Fast Facts About the Historic Connection Between Dental Problems and Chronic Pain

- In Egypt in 3000 B.C., a "dislocation of the mandible" was reported.

- Circa 300 B.C., Hippocrates noted the connection between damaged or crooked teeth and recurring headaches.[7, 10]

- In 1842, Sir Astley Cooper, English surgeon and anatomist, discovered that women may be more prone than men to TMJoint problems, due in part to lowered resistance with abnormal relaxation of joint ligaments.

- Medicine has known since 1914 that the TN is the cranial nerve responsible for chronic migraines when Harry Campbell, M.D., F.R.C.P. wrote his paper titled "Discussion on Headache: Its Causes and Treatment." Campbell explained that the TN is the cranial nerve responsible for chronic migraines, that dental disease is one of the triggers of migraine and recurring daily headaches.[10, 11]

- In 1914, Dr. Campbell noted women were more prone to headaches.

- In 1918, H.J. Prentiss stated that the TMJoint problems became pathologic with the loss of teeth.[12]

- As early as 1934, James Costen M.D. presented findings regarding the connection between the TMJoints, anterior dislocations of the TMJoints, and the irritation or grinding against the auriculotemporal branch of the TNS. He noticed that missing molar support, deep overbites, and dislocations of the TMJoints were associated with the following symptoms: recurring headaches, eye pain, visual symptoms, hearing loss, tinnitus (ringing or noises in the ear), sinus problems, and more.[13] He noted that many of these symptoms were relieved by providing the needed molar support. (Today we have bite computers, EMGs, electromagnetic jaw tracking devices, and MRIs to back up Dr. Costen's findings.)

- In 1958, J. Campbell reported on an eleven-year study[12] of 899 selected cases of temporomandibular arthroses with pain. The study found that 551 of these patients benefited from dental care.

The ratio of females to men was 3.5 to 1 in this study. Treatment was prosthetic in nature, employing a temporary acrylic splint (similar to what we do today in Phase One of therapy) to discover the optimal jaw relations, followed by permanent occlusal reconstruction after close observation over a suitable period of time.

- In 1976, in the second edition of Nathan Shore's book, *Temporomandibular Joint Dysfunction and the Occlusal Equilibration*, the author states, "This disorder is caused by chronic intrinsic micro-trauma within the joint structure itself. Arthrosis is a dysfunction, not a disease, and with proper care and treatment it can be reversed." [13]

- In 1977, Dr. Harold Gelb published a text titled *Clinical Management of Head, Neck, and TMJ Pain and Dysfunction*, as well as a book for the general public called *Killing Pain Without Prescription* in which he describes treatment for headaches and chronic pain.[7]

- Also in 1977, Dr. Lawrence A. Funt and Dr. Brendan C. Stack, Directors for the National Capital Center for Craniofacial Pain, published a document regarding the evolutionary progression of multiple symptoms relative to age and cumulative clinical index pattern correlated from symptoms documented in craniomandibular pain patients.[14] *(See the chart on page 35.)*

If the medical and dental industry had pursued the findings of these men instead of ignoring or covering them up, billions of people through the centuries could have been saved from lifetimes of suffering. NFL players might be wearing red shoes with a "stop chronic pain" logo like they do every October to bring awareness to the need for a cure for breast cancer. We'd be raising awareness and money for the cause of chronic pain prevention and research relative to the TNS and the TMJoints. Instead, everything these men discovered has been squelched and kept under wraps by the Goliaths and dictators of the medical and pharmaceutical companies.

explained that the most common issues to result due to "abnormalities of the teeth" include pain in the head, eyes, neck, arms, and ears. Campbell was unable to find who made the first connection between teeth and headaches—I would submit Hippocrates' connection between crooked teeth and increased headaches as a possible first—but he did credit several authors in the 1700s and 1800s who wrote about the connection. They are: J. Fordyce (1758), Whytt (1765), Stapleton (1777), F. J. Innis (1787), Labarraque (1837), Fabrice de Hilden and Durwin (sic) to the same effect. Also, W. Seller (1848), Symonds (1858), J. Dixon (1856), and S. J. Salter (1868).

Stop for a moment and look at those dates. We are now well into the 2010s. The longevity of this knowledge leaves absolutely no excuse for the medical or dental profession to deny it!

It seems that the problem we have today of the medical and dental professions ignoring the truth about the dental connection to chronic pain isn't a new phenomenon. With all the knowledge available to him, Campbell himself noted, "It is somewhat remarkable that after careful search among the writings of dental surgeons, I have not been able to find any reference to the subject of dental headaches." Isn't it interesting that more than a century later, in the age of dissemination of information, relatively few articles are being written on this topic in the dental journal published by the ADA (American Dental Association)? I have copies and photos of the covers of hundreds of the JADA (Journal of the American Dental Association). Very few, if any, emphasize the suffering of chronic pain patients or how the dental profession can relieve this pain. Yet, the ADA knows it exists! And although a number of dental groups have formed to focus specifically on this chronic problem, in my opinion, it is the ADA's responsibility to educate dental professionals about how imperative it is that they 1) diagnose, 2) do not cause, and

If we don't stop the practice of pain for profit now, it will continue for centuries more.

3) refer suffering patients to qualified dentists for treatment instead of ignoring the issue and allowing the suffering to continue.

The limited number of articles concerning TMD issues that actually make it into *JADA* are rarely cover stories, and are similar to the article in the September 2010 issue titled "Managing the Care of Patients with Temporomandibular Disorders: A New guideline for Care." This allows dentistry and medicine to step backwards and state that TMD problems should be treated as a biopsychosocial problem. This is the "system" throwing the problem back in the patients' laps, blaming them for an inability to cope with life. It opens the door for pharmaceutical companies, medical clinics and hospitals to make hundreds of billions of dollars per year, and never have to examine or refer this to qualified dentists that are able to treat this as the orthopedic neurological problem that it is. I'm not sure if it is the powerful influence of the pharmaceutical industry, or dentistry's fear of admitting their role in stopping and causing chronic pain that allows JADA to avoid hard-hitting articles that could help millions, even billions of people. Do they not realize that there are multiple organizations within dentistry that have formed specifically to deal with treating this epidemic of pain? Dr. H. Clifton Simmons III, D.D.S. wrote a very direct critical review of this biopsychosocial joke to the editor of JADA and they refused to print it. It was however printed in the January 2012 issue of *The Journal of Craniomandibular Practice*.[34]

In the mid-1500s, Andreas Vesalius identified and named the trigeminal nerve system and traced it to teeth.[11] Since that time the medical and dental profession has known that the TNS, which supplies each and every tooth, also supplies both jaw joints and all the muscles involved in chewing and clenching. It's also clear that these muscles, teeth, and jaw joints are connected to the brain by this nerve. Additionally, they are part of the same cranial nerve system, the TNS, that literally surrounds the brain like a canopy and supplies the eyes, ears, sinuses, and much more.

In 1974, I attended a lecture presented by Dr. Harold Gelb. His opening statement struck me and forever changed my perspective on this dental specialty of treating patients with chronic pain. He said, "I've got good news, and I've got bad news. The good news is you are in the best profession in the world for helping people in chronic pain, but you don't even know it. The bad news is it's going to take ten years to filter to the profession, and twenty-five years before it is taught in the dental schools." He understood the medical, pharmaceutical, and even the dental industry's resistance in diagnosing and treating chronic pain with dental origins. I met Dr. Gelb again at a seminar in 2008, and he admitted that the time frame he predicted would almost have to be doubled. My prediction based on the "follow the money" attitude the American healthcare system has adopted is this: If we don't stop the practice of pain for profit now, it will continue for centuries more. The profit machine will become too great and powerful to stop. That's why we're fighting to get this message out. There is no need for this type of suffering to continue at the magnitude at which it does.

IT'S TIME TO CHANGE THE "SYSTEM"

More than enough research, statistics—truths—exist to prove that well-trained dentists can relieve patients of pain caused by recurring assaults on the TNS. Yet, in my office in October 2012, I received a letter from Blue Cross Anthem stating this treatment is experimental. Over the past thirty-eight years that I've been treating this pain, Blue Cross has received progress reports signed by dozens of patients stating that they are 80 to 90 percent better without drugs. Regardless of the marked progress, this insurance company and countless others continue to get away with condemning these patients to suffer for decades longer by denying them coverage. These same patients pay significant monthly insurance premiums to cover their every joint and every nerve in their entire body. Unfortunately, these companies are allowed not to cover one joint and one nerve: the trigeminal nerve system (the largest of the twelve cranial nerves), and the TMJoints. This insurance exclusion forces patients to pay out of pocket for treatment—so most can't afford to have treatment. Years of seeing 80 to 90 percent symptom relief without drugs or surgeries should make insurance excited to cover our treatment. They would actually save hundreds of billions of dollars by covering this relatively inexpensive treatment. Instead, they deny the claims. This lack of foresight begs the question: *Why?* To find the answer, it seems an investigation is in order into who controls these insurance companies' finances.

Major players in the dental profession are aware of this problem. The Wisconsin Dental Association, for example, gave me its full support when I went to the state capitol in 1997 to get the TMJ Bill passed so major medical insurance companies would be forced to cover TMJ as a treatment for chronic migraines, recurring headaches, neck pain, and the list of symptoms. The American Dental Association is also aware that this treatment works. Unfortunately, just as in Harry Campbell's time, only occasional articles are published in the industry's journals about this issue. Worse yet, no initiative has ever been launched to force physicians and dentists to diagnose and refer to specially trained dentists around the world who treat the cause and provide relief without drugs—until now.

The fact that this chronic suffering continues today is a travesty when the medical, dental, insurance, and pharmaceutical industries know full well how to relieve it. In my thirty-eight years of practice, I have seen patient after patient walk through our door and find out for the first time after suffering on a daily basis for ten, twenty, thirty, or even sixty-four years, that a treatment and lasting relief has been available to them for decades. It's heartbreaking to think about how many years of their lives have been lost to pain.

A broken system that ignores scientific evidence and keeps people in pain is the reason we must force dentists and doctors to examine patients for pain caused by assaults on the TNS. We must stand up and demand that this suffering stop! That's why I beg you not to sit on your hands and do nothing. I beg you, and I do this at great risk to myself, but one man alone, even when armed with truth and a very strong faith, cannot defeat a system run by Goliath companies with enormous power and endless financial resources. For real change to occur, it will take everyone showing their outrage and disgust for "The System" that has been responsible for keeping millions in America in pain for the better part of a century.

No, this problem is not in your head, and everyone in the medical, insurance, dental and pharmaceutical company knows it. But if you want justice, if you want insurance companies to be forced to cover treatment, if you want doctors and dentists to—at a minimum—examine and diagnose patients suffering with chronic pain, we must unite and demand that this system change.

THE ANATOMY OF
CHRONIC PAIN

"My life was a living hell before I met Dr. Seymour. I have had excruciating migraines for more than twenty-nine years. As I got older, I developed fibromyalgia, TMJ, and most recently, Trigeminal Neuralgia.

I spent an unfathomable amount of money looking for a way to get rid of the pain, or to find someone who would believe that my pain was real. I have seen countless internal medicine doctors, neurologists, dentists, oral surgeons, TMJ specialists, neurosurgeons, radiation oncologists, acupuncturists, massage therapists, chiropractors, physical therapists, ophthalmologists, and the list goes on.

At one point, I was on more than twenty medications daily just to function! The medications actually made things worse by causing more side effects and rebound pain. By the spring of 2008, I was desperate for relief. I went off the medication and had Gamma Knife surgery. My fifth cranial nerve (trigeminal nerve) was severed at the brain stem with a powerful radiation device. This surgery only caused more side effects, and now I have periods of numbness on the left side of my face. Oh, and the operation cost $60,000.

Shortly after the failed Gamma Knife surgery, a friend of mine introduced me to Dr. Seymour. I was skeptical, but desperate for a normal *life. At my first visit, I was completely comfortable and felt like someone finally understood my pain. My problems were diagnosed very quickly. My TMJoint is permanently dislocated on the right side and dislocates sporadically on the left side. This would explain why 99 percent of my migraines are on the right side of my head. It explains why I had constant migraines, head-neck-shoulder pain, vertigo, ringing in my ears, fatigue, sinus problems, and muscle spasms. Finally, someone had a way to permanently treat it without drugs or surgery. I cried in the chair from relief.*

I got my splint within a week. I felt better immediately. My Trigeminal Neuralgia pain has been gone since."

—**Licensed Therapist and Registered Nurse,**
former chronic pain sufferer

As you can see from this patient's story, the pain associated with the Trigeminal Nerve System and TMJoints extends far beyond the mouth and jaw joints. Fibromyalgia affects nerves throughout the body, as does Trigeminal Neuralgia. In this chapter, I'll explain how this pain travels and why its symptoms are so far reaching. First, though, it may be helpful to understand that there are unique features in the anatomy of the head and neck that enable trained dentists to offer treatment and a cure for chronic pain. This information will give you a better understanding about the source of the symptoms so many people have suffered with for centuries.

The following facts offer insights into why the health of your mouth and jaw are critical to your overall well-being.

- The teeth are the only part of the skeleton that surface anywhere in the body. As such, the skeleton can be permanently altered or balanced without surgery.

46

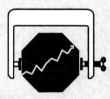

NEWSWORTHY TRUTH

The teeth are the only place in the entire body that the hard support structure of the skeleton is exposed through the skin. It is also the only place where we can permanently change the skeleton without surgery and provide a long-term cure for your pain.

- Your teeth stop the lower jaw from over closing.

- The lower jaw is the only free-hanging bone that crosses the midline in the entire skeleton.

- The upper and lower jaws, as well as every tooth, are supplied by the largest of twelve cranial nerves, the trigeminal nerve system (TNS).

- The lower jaw has two separate joints that, if dislocated, can rub against a branch of the TNS as well as a bone at the base of the brain. Each side of the lower jaw and its TMJoint are controlled by a separate half of the TNS.

- If you are missing certain teeth (support pillars in the skeleton of the head), you are an amputee in the skeleton of the skull.

- The TNS is unique because it is involved in all five senses (sight, hearing, smell, taste, touch) as well as balance.

- The TNS plays an active role in referred pain such as the stabbing eye pain that accompanies migraines, or severe ear pain with no infection, hearing loss, sinus problems, etc.

- The TNS surrounds two-thirds of the brain. It is capable of dictating a forward head posture and curvature of the spine, opening the door for chronic headaches, neck pain, shoulder pain, lower back pain, and vertigo.

- The TNS is unique because it is both a motor and sensory nerve. Most nerves are one or the other. After sensing an irritation the TNS also controls the muscles that go into spasm due to the dislocation.

- Teeth are also unique because they are covered by enamel, the hardest structure in the body. Enamel allows the teeth to withstand extreme forces: hundreds of pounds per square inch (more than most people weigh).

REDEFINING SKELETON AND TEETH

Believe it or not, to get the medical and insurance companies to acknowledge TNS- and TMJ-related pain and the viable treatments available from specially trained dentists, we must first change the definitions of skeleton and tooth.

At present, teeth are not considered part of the skeleton. They are defined in a very limited sense as enamel-coated structures in the jaws used for biting and chewing. The skeleton is defined as the 206 bones in the human body. Those two definitions do not include the fact that the body's thirty-two teeth function as support beams or pillars between the bones in the skeleton of the head and face.

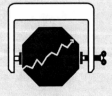

NEWSWORTHY TRUTH

Teeth are used as orthopedic, neurological, structural columns that can alter and eliminate assaults on the TNS and TMJoints in the skeleton of the skull. Teeth must therefore be redefined as **support pillars in the skeleton of the skull.**

Certainly, the teeth are used for biting and chewing. But they serve another, very significant purpose. *The teeth are external, rigid support pillars that function as a framework supporting extreme forces: hundreds of pounds of pressure per square inch when you chew or clench your teeth.* This force is exerted on structures of the skeleton of the skull (the head). If teeth are not vertical support pillars between the bones and the skeleton of the skull, what stops the lower jaw from over closing? What guides it into its final closed position?

Teeth, therefore, must be defined as support pillars in the skeleton of the skull. **Teeth are used as orthopedic, neurological, structural columns that can alter and eliminate assaults on the TNS and TMJoints in the skeleton of the skull.** The definition of teeth and skeleton should also include the fact that teeth, the bones of the jaw, chewing muscles, and jaw joints are all supplied by a nerve that literally surrounds the brain like a canopy.

You may ask why it is so important to correct the definitions of the teeth and skeleton. Consider this: Anyone who is missing teeth, particularly molars, is essentially an "amputee" in the skeleton of the skull. Once removed, human extremities do not grow back. Transplants, implants, or prostheses are the only options for recovering the loss of an amputated limb, or extracted tooth. Over time, the absence of these essential support structures (the teeth) causes stress, damage, discomfort, or significant pain. Because the teeth are the only place in the entire body where the hard support structure of the skeleton is exposed through the skin, it is also the only place where we can permanently change the skeleton without surgery and provide a long-term cure for your pain.

If the medical, dental, and insurance industries are forced to acknowledge the true definitions of teeth and skeleton, they will also be forced to recognize the importance of the teeth to a person's well-being. However as it stands, amputees of the skull (people who are missing teeth) do not receive proper treatment. The medical community as a whole denies (or ignores) the amount of pressure the teeth withstand as well as their necessary function as support pillars in the skull. One common sense question to ask about the current, limited definition of teeth is: Why are they covered with enamel, the hardest structure in the entire body, if they are not designed to handle extreme pressure?

THE TRIPLANE COMFORT POSITION: FINDING YOUR "HAPPY PLACE"

One of the primary functions of the teeth is to stop the closure of the mouth at a specific desired height. They guide the impact and bring the two arches of teeth together in an ideal position relative to the triplane of comfort. Let me take a moment here to explain the triplane comfort position. The lower jaw is the moving part and it has an ideal position right to left (the sagittal plane), front to back (frontal plane,) and up and down (horizontal plane).

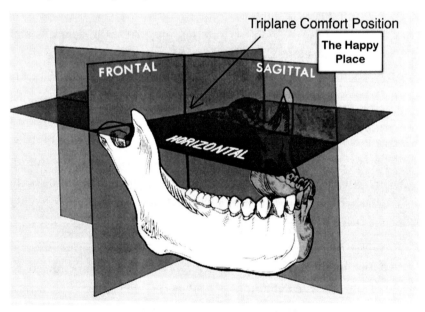

The Triplane Comfort Position (Happy Place) is that sagittal, frontal, and horizontal point where the lower jaw, both jaw joints, and powerful clenching muscles no longer irritate the TNS. A clear plastic, removable lower orthotic is used to locate this position. Only when we are able to prove it's possible to eliminate the pain with the orthotic do we offer the long-term cure of permanently altering the teeth to that position in Phase Two.

When teeth are extracted, crooked, worn down, or missing and not replaced, the remaining teeth shift, and the final closure position is antagonistic to all three planes. The triplane comfort position, or the "Happy Place" as one our patients named it, is now forced into an unhappy position every time the teeth collide in final closure or function to chew, clench, or grind.

To understand the discomfort throughout the muscles, bones, teeth, joints and nerves of the skeleton of the skull when the support pillars (teeth) are out of alignment, imagine bending your arm to lift a dumbbell in a curling motion, your bicep muscle bulging with the effort. The correct way to lift the weight is straight up without turning the wrist. But what if, at the final second of the curling motion, you grab the fist of the curling hand with the opposite hand and twist and twist it away from your body? That movement would be uncomfortable even on the first action. And if this torquing movement were repeated hundreds of times per day, that discomfort would shift to actual pain. Can you see how over time this would trigger pain in your wrist, forearm muscles, bicep, and eventually in your elbow and shoulder?

Patients whose upper and lower arches of teeth do not mesh perfectly (crooked teeth or class II or III malocclusion), experience similar unnatural and uncomfortable glancing movements hundreds

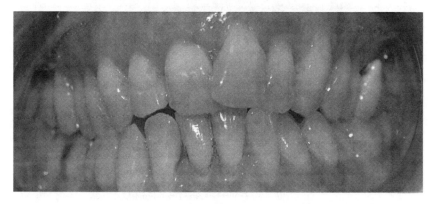

An example of crooked/misaligned teeth

to thousands of times each day at the last second of closure. We must remember that this occurs at hundreds of pounds of pressure per square inch, which is more than you weigh, in the back of the mouth.

I can speak personally about being an amputee of the skeleton of the skull without replacements, fixed bridges or implants. I came from a low-income family in the Upper Peninsula of Michigan, and later, the inner city of Milwaukee, Wisconsin. My six-year molars were extracted (amputated) when I was a teenager. No root canals were done in our neighborhood, and I can remember only one kid who had braces in my high school.

Unbeknownst to me, my second molars collapsed and went into crossbite, the opposite of the ideal alignment that they should have. My triplane support was misaligned and therefore did not properly align my final or second closure. I was constantly stretching my chewing muscles. I often hid my mouth with my hands to cover the imperfections. Aside from my cross bite, I had very sensitive teeth. By the time I was accepted into dental school at age twenty-one, my lower jaw was being displaced relative to all three of those planes every time my teeth came together. In dental school, I heard, for the first time, from a dentist, that I needed bridges and extensive dental work; but nothing was mentioned about

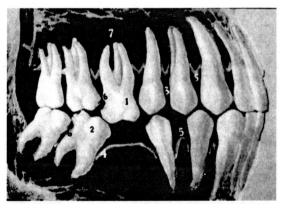

When molars are extracted (amputated) and not replaced, the triplane support becomes misaligned.

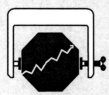

NEWSWORTHY TRUTH

Over closure on one side of your mouth and a less-than-ideal balance relative to the triplane comfort position not only affects beauty and facial symmetry, over closure also has an effect on athletic performance, singing, and the playing of many musical instruments. These joints and muscles are in constant use.

the triplane comfort position and no one asked if I suffered from chronic pain. Although I did not experience migraines, I had occasional headaches and frequent neck and shoulder tightness and pain. Neither I nor my professors thought to associate my collapsed bite and dislocated TMJoints with this pain.

From my own experience as an amputee of the skeleton of the skull, I can relate to people who have this problem and no one so much as tells them about it. If you are missing all the molars on one side of your mouth, it's like having your leg cut off at the knee. You truly are an amputee in the skeleton of the skull. The side of your mouth with teeth will stop when the teeth come into contact, but on the other side of your mouth with missing teeth, the jaw will over close, compressing the condyle (the ball portion of the lower jaw) of the TMJ against the bone at the base of the brain and against the front wall of your ear hundreds of times a day. Doctors will automatically recommend a prosthesis for a leg amputee, so why don't they recommend the equivalent procedure for a person with missing molars? Without an accurate prosthesis nothing will stop your lower jaw from over closing on the affected side.

The way your teeth provide proper support, the way they mesh, and the way they guide or stop your jaw closing is key to the structural symmetry of your head and face. When the upper and lower jaws don't align properly facial symmetry and beauty are affected: one eye opens more than the other, muscles develop on one side more than the other, and wrinkles and sunken cheeks develop on the other side. Head and shoulder posture will follow suit.

IS YOUR BODY TRYING TO AVOID PAIN?

Missing teeth, along with sensitive, broken-down, fractured, uneven, and crooked teeth act like a stone in your shoe. If you have a rock in your shoe, do you have the option not to limp? No. The number one reflex in the body, the "avoidance of pain" reflex, forces you to limp to avoid even the tiniest pebble. It's so uncomfortable, that most people will immediately stop what they're doing to remove the source of the irritation. Soon after the stone is removed, the pain dissipates as well.

But what happens if you continued to walk with a stone in your shoe for years? Beyond developing a sore where the rock presses into the skin, the awkwardness of the limp will eventually cause soreness in your legs, hips and back.

The same thing happens in your mouth due to the avoidance of pain reflex. Uneven, broken, or missing teeth eventually cause stress on the remaining teeth, bones, muscles, and joints. You reflexively avoid the sensitive tooth, dislocated TMJoint, or the side with no teeth. This "limp" causes a chain reaction of pain and explains why the "pain anxiety cycle" regenerates itself day in and day out for decades.

Let's use clenching during sleep as a simple example to explain the never-ending "pain anxiety cycle." If your teeth are out of alignment and one or both of your TMJoints are dislocated, the muscles surrounding this joint will go into spasm while you're sleeping in an effort to prevent the dislocated joint from over compressing against the branch of the TNS that passes through the TMJoint. Throughout the night, you will—to no avail—continually, yet unconsciously, clench and grind your teeth in an effort to make your bite fit (or align). Every morning, you will

> *The number one reflex in the body, the "avoidance of pain"*
> *reflex, forces you to limp to avoid even the tiniest pebble.*

wake up exhausted, unrested, and in pain. Enamel is the hardest structure in the body. It takes years to grind it in. So, night after night, the same clenching and grinding occurs, keeping the pain anxiety cycle in motion. This phenomenon recycles pain for years and decades, which means doctors often have ample time to recognize the problem. Yet, the entire medical community is permitted not to look or examine you for a dislocated TMJoint. *Try to think of another joint in the body that if dislocated no one cares.* There simply isn't one.

Meanwhile, the TMJoints are essential for life and are used thousands of time a day. *They never get to rest,* and they are supplied by and have the power to trigger pain in a nerve that surrounds the brain. Why are doctors permitted to ignore these two joints? Oh, that's right, "follow the money."

The pain-avoidance reflex also allows a trained dentist to cure your pain. Using a bite computer and a custom orthotic with guidance systems it is possible to locate the triplane comfort position, the "happy place," where the TNS is no longer in hyper-response mode. If we eliminate or significantly reduce the multiple traumatic assaults on the TNS, we are able to stop the muscle's spasms and reduce compression and swelling in the temporomandibular joints. Just as removing a stone from your shoe, when we eliminate the assaults on the TNS—assaults that can come from misaligned or missing teeth, muscles that are in spasm or are swollen, bone growth or anomalies, dislocated joints—the pain goes away, and more importantly stays away!

This reflex is the number one reflex in the body, a protection mode programed into the nervous system to call attention to areas of the body that are being traumatized or injured. In essence it is a warning system that screams, "Help me! Get rid of this trauma!" It certainly doesn't scream, "Cover me up and mask me with drugs so I can keep being hurt over and over again." No, the reflex is there to notify you of the problem so the cause can be addressed before it does irreparable damage.

UNDERSTANDING THE TEMPOROMANDIBULAR JOINTS

The TMJoints lie at the base of the brain on either side of the head. I mentioned earlier that this problem is much more extensive than the catch-all diagnosis of TMJ. That said, the importance of the TMJoints cannot be disregarded. They are essential to your well-being and as such they never get to rest, even when they are dislocated or arthritic because they are essential to life. Below is a partial list of when TMJoints are used:

- Speaking
- Singing
- Biting
- Licking
- Eating
- Swallowing
- Mouth breathing
- Sleeping (clenching, grinding)
- Yawning
- Coughing
- Crying
- Laughing
- Vomiting
- Chewing gum
- Blowing bubbles
- Intimacy

- Whistling
- Playing musical instruments

When the TMJoints are dislocated, displaced, or arthritic, those simple life activities irritate these joints to the max.

During weather changes, dislocated or arthritic jaw joints react just like other arthritic joints due to barometric pressure drops. Because the joints are already swollen, when the barometric pressure drops, the pressure in the stressed joints doesn't immediately equalize with atmospheric pressure. Instead, they expand more, putting additional pressure on the trigeminal nerve (TN). The end result is increased pain as storms roll in.

When the TMJoints are dislocated or arthritic, the powerful muscles surrounding these joints go into spasm. These muscle spasms can also trigger the complex TN, particularly the auriculotemporal branch of the TNS, which runs to the condyle between the ear and the condyle of the mandible. This means the auriculotemporal branch of the TNS gets pinched between the bone at the floor of the brain that makes up the fossa and condyle (the ball portion of the joint). The action is similar to chalking a pool cue, with the extremely sensitive nerve caught in the middle.

Why is a joint that lies against the floor of the brain, that never gets to rest because it is used in so many vital functions, and is often dislocated or arthritic, not of interest to anyone in the medical community? It doesn't make sense! In the self-exam and survey (Chapter Five) you will likely discover that you have never been examined for a dislocated or arthritic jaw joint. If you suffer from chronic migraines, tension headaches, back pain, ear pain, or any of the other types of pain listed in Chapter One, this should be one of the first places doctors and dentists look. The joints are very easy to examine because they are close to the surface of the skin, right in front of your ears.

Speaking of ears, patients with dislocated, inflamed, or arthritic TMJoints sometimes experience hearing loss, ringing in the ears, or stabbing ear pain. There are two key reasons for this. First, the swelling of the TMJoint, which is only two millimeters from the ear, can put pressure on the eustachian tube and ear canal. Second, a direct branch of the TNS is attached to the tensor tympani muscle that controls the tension on the eardrum. The name speaks for itself. The tension on the surface of a tympani drum in an orchestra is altered by the amount of pressure or tightness of that surface. The same principle holds true in regard to the eardrum. In this way, the TMJoints and the TNS cause a symptom that too many physicians ignore and misdiagnose.

As I mentioned in the introduction, this isn't simply about "TMJ." The pain these joints can trigger extends far beyond the mouth and jaw because of their connection to the trigeminal nerve system.

UNDERSTANDING THE TRIGEMINAL NERVE SYSTEM

The far-reaching effects of the trigeminal nerve system (TNS) are much greater than "TMJ," a phrase that has become a catch-all term. Because of the major role it plays in the body, the TNS could very well be a key alarm system to the prevention of chronic pain, sleep loss, poor posture, decreased energy levels, strength, and balance, as well as chronic fatigue and chronic depression. The TNS surrounds the mainframe hard drive of the central nervous system, and it is called the chief sensory nerve of the head and face. The medical and dental world should be forced to view this nerve system with the importance it deserves, as a highly sensitive alarm, rather than tuning it out with drugs. *Paying attention to its obvious warnings could lead to the prevention of many health problems, drug addictions, hearing loss, back pain, and many needless surgeries throughout life.* But if no one looks and the alarm is simply ignored, people will continue to be robbed of their quality of life for years or decades.

Look at the other major structures they supply to see why the TNS and dislocated TMJoints compressing against and irritating a nerve system of this magnitude are capable of causing so many far-reaching symptoms. This major, cranial nerve system is involved in some way with all five senses, as well as the sense of balance. It supplies the eyes,

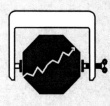

NEWSWORTHY TRUTH

Because of the major role it plays in the body, the TNS could very well be a key alarm system to the prevention of chronic pain, sleep loss, poor posture, increased energy levels, strength, balance, as well as chronic fatigue and chronic depression.

ears, sinuses, tongue, throat, the jaw joints (temporomandibular joints), neck, and chewing muscles. This is why it is called the chief sensory nerve of the head and face. The TNS receives input from the eyes, ears, tongue, and brainstem, and accounts for 50 percent of the information that enters the brain. Exactly how is the medical community permitted to ignore assaults on a nerve of this importance? Again "follow the money."

The TNS can refer recurring pain symptoms throughout this extensive nerve system and far beyond. The reason it refers pain to joints down the entire body has to do with the stone in the shoe analogy. If you limp long enough you'll develop ankle pain, knee pain, hip pain, and back pain. An assault on the TNS in the form of a dislocated or arthritic TMJoint, or sensitive, misaligned, or missing teeth, will cause a "limp" in the mouth. Eventually, your head posture will shift. The weight of the head being off center when combined with the continual pull of gravity changes the functional engineering and stress on every weight-bearing joint in your neck, back, hips, knees, and ankles. Even your toes must do extra work to keep you upright!

Most nerves are either sensory and detect pain, touch, heat, cold, etc., or they are motor nerves that control muscle movement. The TN is one of a few nerves that is both sensory and motor. The motor portion supplies all the muscles of mastication, your clenching, chewing, and grinding muscles, including the masseter muscle, the strongest muscle in the body. This group of muscles also includes the huge temporalis muscle I've mentioned that lies directly over the temple where many headaches and migraines occur.

A ROAD MAP OF SYMPTOMS

By now it should be evident that the encompassing nature of the TNS makes it a unique and critical structure in the human body. You can also see how pain that begins in the mouth can be referred to other areas of the body. The reality is that pain symptoms travel the three branches of the trigeminal nerve system like a road map. Here is a brief list of general symptoms that are directly related to the trigeminal nerve system (TNS), or indirectly related through referred pain or forced changes in the posture of the head, neck and shoulders in response to the avoidance of pain reflex irritations or trauma to the TNS.

Neuralgia

This means acute stimulated or provoked pain radiating along the course of one or more nerves usually without demonstrable changes in the nerve structure. With neuralgias of the TNS, the pain follows the nerve throughout the head, face, and neck.

Atypical trigeminal neuralgia

The symptoms of atypical neuralgia (ATN) tend to be vague and misleading. As such, ATN may be the most misdiagnosed form of neuralgia. The symptoms can be mistaken for migraines, dental problems such as TMJ, muscular and skeletal issues. Physicians often blame the symptoms on hypochondria, basically saying, "It's all in your head."

Indeed, this pain really is all in the head as it relates to the muscles, joints and nerves associated with the skeleton of the head and the TNS, but it is not psychological or imagined. The TNS controls the muscles you use to open and close your mouth, to chew, and to clench your teeth all night—the muscles of mastication. It controls the huge temporalis muscle over your temples where many of your headaches appear. Like the stone in the shoe that forces you to favor one foot or the other, irritations via the teeth, muscles, bones, and joints of the TNS will force you to chew on one side more than the other. This imbalance causes poor head posture (forward and off to one side) resulting in headaches that come up from the back of the neck, as well as the neck aches. Eventually, the unnatural head posture leads to rounded shoulders and more forward weight distribution that causes a chain reaction of strain on weight-bearing joints like the lower back, hips, and knees down the entire body. When you think about it, your toes have to be working harder to keep you upright.

That's enough about general symptoms referred far away from the TNS. Now let's look specifically at some of the chronic life-altering physical symptoms related to the TNS.

Headaches

These are chronic, recurring headaches, migraines, stress (tension), sinus, cluster and morning headaches located in the temple areas, on top of the head, and those that come up from the neck and back of the head.

Sleep loss

Intense forces are induced during the clenching and bruxing that occur during sleep. This triggers the trigeminal nerve all night long, and deeper levels of REM sleep are not achieved because pain is generated during sleep. Headaches and other symptoms frequently occur night after night, and it's almost impossible to get your head off the pillow in the morning.

Sleep apnea

This is an intermittent cessation of breathing during sleep. The TNS and the alignment of your bite will dictate how far back your lower jaw positions itself. Try this experiment: Pull back your lower jaw and breathe through your nose or mouth. Notice how labored your breathing is when your jaw is pulled back. It's like pinching off or constricting your airway. The airway is basically a tube with a flap of cartilage over it. That flap, called the epiglottis, seals off the airway from food. When your jaw falls back too far during sleep, it can inhibit airflow. A trained dentist could move your jaw forward with a nocturnal appliance and get you off that CPAP (a breathing assist device with a mask and tubes hooked up to an oxygen tank) and sleeping well again.

Eye symptoms

These are extreme pressure and stabbing pain behind the eye, aura, light sensitivity, dry eye or excessive tearing. Patients describe this pain as an "ice pick" or "hot poker" in the eye. The TNS regulates the aqueous humor fluid pressure in the eye, shaping the cornea and the lens. It also controls how rapidly the pupil dilates or contracts, as well as the functioning of the lacrymal gland that produces tears.

Trigeminal neuralgia or tic douloureux

This is extreme facial pain described as sudden, sharp, stabbing or burning, and severe, that follows the path of the trigeminal nerve. Remember the two largest branches, the maxillary and mandibular branches of the TNS, are very commonly chronically irritated or under attack by poorly aligned teeth, missing teeth, dislocated TMJoints, and muscle spasms caused by the dislocated joints.

Vertigo

This dizziness can make it difficult to walk or drive. The forward head posture, looking down at the pavement versus up at the horizon plays a role here. We are able to eliminate vertigo and dizziness in nine out of ten cases without drugs.

Ear symptoms

These are sharp shooting pain, tinnitus, hearing loss, inability to clear ears by swallowing, and pain with no infection.

Teeth

The malposed teeth often become sensitive, leading to needless root canals, fractured teeth, extractions, costly bridges or implants, gum disease, bone loss, etc. The TNS is extremely sensitive and enamel is the hardest substance in the human body. As the nerve that supplies the teeth, the TNS can detect high spots in the bite when opposing enamel collides as small as 1/10,000th of a millimeter—that's the equivalent of 1/1000th of the thickness of an average strand of human hair. If you've ever had a crown or filling built too high, you may remember the pain this nerve registered to not only that tooth, but to the ear, and possibly the entire side of your face.

Sinuses

Symptoms may mimic sinusitis; increased mucous production, and post-nasal drip. Antibiotics do nothing, and numerous patients have had needless sinus surgery over this.

Neck pain

It occurs due to the forward or lateral (scoliosis) head posture these patients often develop trying to favor one side or the other in their bite due to dislocated TMJoints, teeth that are being repeatedly traumatized, or muscle spasms in the chewing muscles. The head weighs as much as a bowling ball and is not exempt from gravity, causing muscles in the neck and throughout the body to go into spasm trying to compensate. The pain moves down the body and causes the following...

Fibromyalgia & back pain

Tenderness or general pain in the muscles, joints, tendons and other soft tissues. Aches in the shoulders, upper and lower back.

Temporomandibular joint pain

Clicking and popping within the jaw joints (TMJs) indicate dislo-cated discs within the joints causing limited opening, inflammation and swelling in the joints, and bone-on-bone crepitus or grating sounds during opening and closing. A branch of the TNS is usually being repeatedly crushed or ground against in these situations, like a pool cue being chalked, referring pain all over the head, neck and rest of the body.

Muscle spasms

Muscles of the head and face spasm like muscles in the back if the disc is displaced or a nerve is being rubbed on or irritated between two vertebrae.

Drugs are not the answer to these problems. In truth, drugs only mask the symptoms, cloud the patient's mental clarity, and create long-term side effects, systemic complications and loss of teeth due to covering up or masking the cause.

Now that you have a better understanding of how these physical structures work, we'll take a look at how TNS- and TMJ-related pain disproportionately affect women, the elderly and the poor.

The Truth About the Female Epidemic of Chronic Pain and Migraines

THROUGHOUT HER TWENTIES AND THIRTIES, PEOPLE CONSTANTLY TOLD SUE SHE LOOKED EXHAUSTED... AND SHE WAS. Dealing with the pain she experienced on a daily basis put her in "survival mode." She tried every remedy she could think of to get rid of her debilitating headaches; she even went to an acupuncturist three times a week for temporary relief. "But that wasn't a cure. No medication helped. It was absolutely debilitating, like a hot poker in my right eye. Once it started it would go on for an entire week. I don't know how I survived when I look back now," Sue says. "Dating was not even on my radar screen. I was going to work and that was about it."

Sue found her way to my office in her mid-forties. We quickly found the temporary solution for her bite issues that stemmed from crooked teeth and a small mouth. Using a split, we were able to relieve the pain.

"I was so thankful for that change, that elimination of the daily pain," she says. She felt better and was finally able to enjoy life. She even started dating and got engaged. "After the splint had proved what it was able to do, my fiancé and I realized I needed to go ahead with the permanent dental work. It was then I felt we could actually plan a wedding."

For years, the intense pain had kept Sue from fully living. She even put off getting married. Her fear: "What if I got one of those horrific headaches on that day? I wouldn't be able to attend my own wedding." She had also never considered having children. "I could barely take care of myself let alone take care of someone else. Since I've gotten rid of the pain, we got a dog. I wouldn't even have been able to have had a pet prior to this," she says.

"Chronic pain is debilitating. The headaches were profound. Now, my life is profound. I get up in the morning without headache. I can turn on the radio. I can sit down and have breakfast and listen to the news or pick up the paper and read. I can go to work and not be in pain. But the biggest change is just being able to come home from work, walk the dog, cook a meal, and enjoy the evening. I love that I no longer live in the constant fear that the pain will come back."

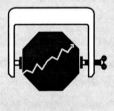

NEWSWORTHY TRUTH

While the system refuses to offer real relief it charges patients hundreds of billions of dollars each year for testing, unneeded surgeries, drugs to cover up the real problem, and repeated treatments that only offer temporary relief.

Can you imagine what it would feel like to live without chronic pain? Many women can't. They suffer daily with headaches, backaches, neck pain, and a host of other physical, mental and emotional symptoms that for centuries the medical profession has blamed on hormones. And what doctors can't chalk up to hormones they blame on women's inability to cope with life. Drugs—pain relievers, hormones, muscle relaxers, anti-depressants, and other fog-inducing pharmaceuticals—are prescribed to mask chronic, recurrent pain. Meanwhile, the true cause goes untreated, ultimately perpetuating an unrelenting cycle of suffering. The medical community's practice of simply ignoring the TNS and TMJ is infuriating and shameful. Adding insult to injury, while the system refuses to offer real relief it **charges patients hundreds of billions of dollars**[34, 36] **each year for testing, unneeded surgeries, drugs to cover up the real problem, and repeated treatments that only offer temporary relief.** The truth is there are a number of issues that are more likely than hormones to cause chronic pain, migraines, and tension headaches. It should be clear now that when we address the cause of pain, it is possible to eliminate the painful symptoms. In the previous chapter you learned about the trigeminal nerve system (TNS) and its role in any number of types of chronic pain. In the introduction I noted that women are disproportionately affected by TNS- and TMJ-related migraines, tension headaches, and a number of other chronic pain symptoms.

This chapter will help you understand why with several **Newsworthy Truths about chronic pain as it relates specifically to women.** You'll learn:

- Why women are **three times** more likely than men to suffer from migraines, fibromyalgia, and numerous other symptoms associated with chronic pain,

- That painful symptoms have been **mistakenly blamed on hormones for centuries,**

- How the same **structural, neurological, and muscular imbalances** that cause the pain **also affect beauty and facial symmetry,**

- That chronic pain can also damage **self-esteem and relationships,**

- Why **women must unite to stop the abuse** they're subjected to by the current medical system.

Why Women Suffer from Chronic Pain Three Times More Frequently than Men

Let's take a look at the first truth—the one about which my wife says, "If men comprised the majority of chronic pain suffers, a cure would be readily available and covered by insurance!" The truth: *75 percent of patients with TMJ-related pain are women.*[3, 7, 12] 75 percent! The study that revealed this truth also found that women are five times[4] more likely than men to have TMJ disk displacement. The findings indicate that women are more sensitive to pain conditions, reporting more severe pain, more frequent pain, and pain of longer duration than men. Although the study's ratio for TMJ-related pain was three to one, at the Chronic Pain Solution Center we treat eight women for every man.

A number of factors account for this disparity of pain between women and men. Let's start with the fact that women are five times more likely to have a dislocated TMJ.[4] Why? One reason is that women have smaller mouths and are thus more likely to have crooked or crowded teeth. (Men, I can't tell you how difficult it was for me to admit that women have smaller mouths, please don't hold it against me. We are going to get rid of their headaches... that should be worth something.) In general, women have petite skulls with smaller dental arches. The size of a person's dental arch and skull is obviously dependent on genetics and ethnicity, but compared to men, women's mouths are smaller. Having smaller dental arches means there is less room for the same number of teeth. In a melting pot like the United States where people of different ethnic groups and nationalities frequently intermarry, this problem is exacerbated. When a woman with small dental arches inherits Dad's or Grandpa's teeth from an ethnic group that is known to have large arches and large teeth, there simply isn't room in her mouth. This is one reason that more women than men have crowded teeth.

Our bodies are designed to allow teeth to erupt through the gum tissue in an orderly manner. When a dental arch is too small and there is not enough room, the teeth automatically rotate to fit the narrow space. The result is crooked and misaligned teeth that don't mesh with the opposing arch of teeth causing the displacement of the lower jaw and both TMJoints.

As you read earlier in this book, historical studies verify the connection between crooked teeth and chronic headaches and neck pain. More than 2,500 years ago, Hippocrates noted[7, 10] that people with crooked teeth are more likely to experience recurring headaches. Hippocrates' findings were not exclusive or specific to women, but a number of more recent studies have found that crooked teeth are more prevalent in women. A European research group studied the bites of approximately 200,000 men and women and found that 70 percent of women have a malocclusion (an imperfect bite) compared to men. The researchers considered a bite to have a malocclusion if the person had at least one rotated tooth.

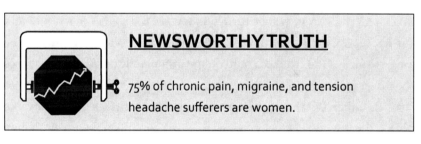

NEWSWORTHY TRUTH

75% of chronic pain, migraine, and tension headache sufferers are women.

Remember, the human body is not exempt from the laws of physics, simple machines, and structural engineering. Like a very sophisticated machine, the body is designed to move and operate in a specific manner. Ideally, the teeth of the upper and lower arches should line up and mesh together perfectly like finely-tuned gears on a clock or a transmission of a car. Imagine mechanical gears on a clock or on a transmission coming together to function, but the notches are offset and the teeth are missing, crooked, or otherwise out of alignment. Would you expect that clock to keep accurate time? Would you take the car on a long trip… if it could run at all? Certainly not! The result of crowded teeth is that the upper and lower arches of teeth cannot mesh together precisely.

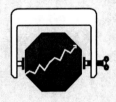

NEWSWORTHY TRUTH

Hormones are **not** the most likely cause of women's chronic pain and migraines.

Most often it's the front teeth rotating to fit into the smaller arch form. The front teeth are particularly important because they provide the guidance systems that dictate the final position front to back (frontal plane) which the lower jaw will be forced into on closing. When a lower front tooth is rotated, one corner of that tooth is popped forward more than the natural outer curvature of the lower dental arch. Each time the jaw closes, this poorly aligned tooth strikes the back of the inside surface of the upper front teeth that don't move. If it is an upper front tooth that is rotated, one corner will be turned in toward the roof of the mouth and further back than it should be. Upon closure, the bottom teeth strike the back surface of the crooked tooth on the immovable upper jaw and force the lower jaw back.

In either instance, when a movable object strikes an immovable object, the movable object gives way. In the case of cooked teeth, when the movable lower jaw strikes the immovable upper jaw, the lower jaw gives way; it is forced back or off to one side. This action forces the lower jaw, *both temporal mandibular joints,* the entire lower arch of teeth, and the most powerful muscles in the body to function farther toward the back of the skeleton of the skull than they were designed to function. The temporal mandibular joints operate on a disc that is designed to move forward and up, centered in the fossa of the joint. When crooked teeth push the jaw back, the TMJoints are forced into an unnatural position that can lead to irritation, swelling, and dislocation.

Simple mechanics explain some of the 5:1 ratio of TMJ disc displacement in women versus men. We have had numerous patients at the Chronic Pain Solution Center who have come to us after suffering for twenty to forty years. Most of these women had clicking, popping, or grating in the joints, a clear sign that the joint could be dislocated. The medical and insurance industries and even some dentists are content to ignore a dislocated or inflamed TMJ and treat it as if it's of no importance. *Nowhere else in the body is a dislocated joint considered unimportant!* If men were five times as likely to have this joint dislocated, do you think the medical profession would still be ignoring it? Dislocated TMJoints are not only painful, they perpetuate the myth that hormones are the primary cause of migraines and other recurring pain. Which brings us to the next point: Hormones are not to blame for the majority of migraines and chronic pain.

WHY HORMONES ARE MISTAKENLY BLAMED FOR CHRONIC PAIN — ESPECIALLY MIGRAINES

No direct evidence exists to link reproductive hormones to TMJ-related pain. In fact, rather than relieving symptoms, commonly prescribed hormone treatments can actually increase the intensity of the pain if nothing is done to eliminate the numerous irritations to the TNS. My purpose here is not to explain hormones, but to share why the cause of the pain many women endure has been mistaken for hormones for centuries.

Pain and swelling occur in any dislocated joint in the body. It stands to reason that the swelling and inflammation that accompany TMJ dislocations are compounded by the fluid retention that occurs during a woman's cycle. When an already swollen, dislocated TMJ endures even greater pressure caused by bloating, the effect is increased irritation of the branch of the TNS that passes through the back of the TMJ. Hormones aren't causing the pain; the swelling and increased pressure in an irritated or dislocated joint (or joints) is the cause of the pain.

Here's the good news: If we eliminate the compression in the joint by increasing the height of the teeth with a custom, plastic orthotic, the swelling of the joint is significantly reduced. Then, when hormones increase the fluid retention within the joint, it doesn't cause that horrific pain many women have come to expect during their cycles. **This should be very exciting news for women who have had everything from chronic headaches to chronic fatigue and depression blamed on hormones since puberty. Imagine eliminating the headache pain and irritability associated with PMS and the monthly cycle. How much could that change your relationships at home and at your place of employment?** This is a huge newsworthy truth, one of the biggest in the whole book, and I've never seen it anywhere in print before. This news alone is world-changing!

Speaking of puberty, the onset of womanhood is often when young ladies begin experiencing migraines. The undeniable timing is another reason hormones are blamed for these debilitating headaches. Earlier in this book, I proposed another perspective on the cause of many types of chronic pain, migraines, and tension headaches—and it has nothing to do with hormones. At about the same time that puberty and hormones enter the picture in a young woman's life, the twelve-year molars and upper cuspid teeth (also known as eye teeth or canines) surface. Those upper and lower cuspids are the most important teeth in the entire

NEWSWORTHY TRUTH

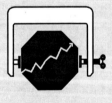

If we eliminate the compression in the joint by increasing the height of the teeth with a custom, plastic orthotic, the swelling of the joint is significantly reduced. Then, when hormones increase the fluid retention within the joint, it doesn't cause that horrific pain many women have come to expect during their cycles.

mouth for the guidance necessary to prevent chronic interferences on the twelve-year molars during chewing and lateral movements of the lower jaw.

Here is a more complete explanation as to why the cuspids and twelve-year molars are capable of not only causing these horrific headaches and other symptoms, but more importantly it explains why this pain recurs, day after day over the course of years or even decades of life. The upper and lower cuspids are specially designed with longer roots to enable them to absorb the lateral (side-to-side) forces during the chewing and grinding movements of the mouth. The cuspids are the cornerstones of the arches. They have the very important function of guiding the lower jaw to close properly relative to the right to left plane (sagittal plane). If a young woman's front teeth are crowded and the cuspids are not brought into proper position with orthodontic treatment, they will not provide the necessary clearance between upper and lower twelve-year molars. If the cuspids are not perfectly aligned, the pointed cusp tips of these new twelve-year molars in the back of the lower arch of teeth will repeatedly bump into or collide with the opposing twelve-year molar during side-to-side chewing or right and left grinding movements at night during sleep in an effort to grind down these interferences. The result is a terrible headache, morning after morning, for decades.

Now pair this information with the illustration I gave earlier about the forces in the bite functioning similar to a nutcracker. The closer you get to the joint of the nutcracker, the more powerful the lever mechanics. The physics of that simple machine multiply the force and enable you to easily crack the nut. In the mouth, the TMJ and your twelve-year molars, are the most powerful parts of your nutcracker. At twelve to fourteen years old these molars are as far back as you can get. At eighteen the wisdom teeth, or third molars, come in—or don't come in properly due to lack of room—and present a whole new set of problems that can generate recurring pain.

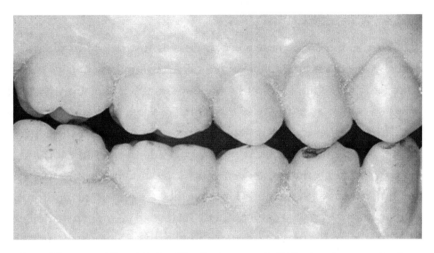

FIG. 1: When a cuspid is pointed and functioning properly, the back molars separate when they chew or grind teeth to the right.

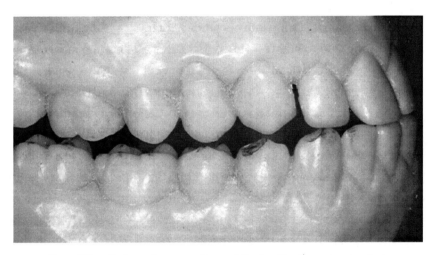

FIG. 2: When the lower jaw moves forward, the front teeth cause separation in the back of the mouth.

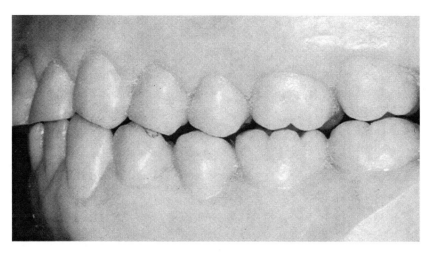

Fig. 3: If eye teeth are worn flat, the back molars do not lift off. This can trigger a lifetime of headaches.

If the upper and lower canine teeth do not guide the two arches of pointed steep cusps and valleys of the lower molars to separate (See Fig. 4, p. 78.) and clear the same type of pointed, convoluted, steep cusp tips of the upper molars immediately during chewing and side-to-side grinding movements, it is like the lower jaw is being forced to grind right and left over speed bumps at extreme forces of hundreds of pounds per square inch. In contrast, if the cuspids are in the proper position, the lower cuspid will immediately contact and glide up the inside, smooth enamel surface of the upper cuspid. The lower jaw will then glide on a nice, smooth surface. In essence, the lower molars will clear the speed bumps of the upper molars and slide along as if gliding on ice, not going through gymnastics and uncomfortable movements in an effort to get over the speed bumps.

If the twelve-year molars or wisdom teeth continually interfere with each other in lateral movements because the cuspids don't provide the necessary clearance, the body's remedy is to attempt to grind those

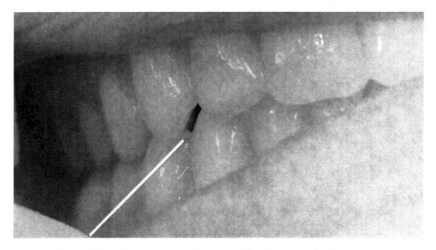

FIG. 4: This patient's upper and lower cuspids miss contacting by 1.5 mm, creating massive interferences on the 12-year molars. (See FIG. 4a below.)

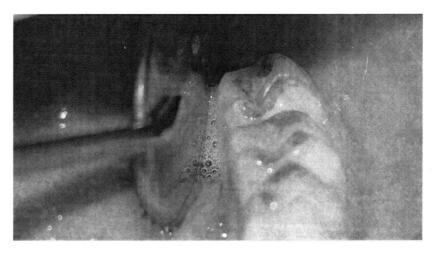

FIG. 4a: The dark spots on the back molars reveal the interferences caused by the 1.5 mm gap above.

irritating interferences down. Of course this grinding doesn't happen during the day, but at night, when hundreds of pounds of pressure per square inch are exerted on the teeth. At the same time, the TNS and both TMJ are being compressed and irritated. In turn, the uncomfortable disjointed movements and extreme pressure prevent the person from reaching the deeper REM (rapid eye movement) levels of sleep. When this goes on for years, it leads to chronic fatigue and depression that stem from waking up in pain day after day. This is also what causes what's referred to as the "pain anxiety cycle."

Pain anxiety cycle: the name alone indicates that doctors want patients to believe that their anxiety is the root cause of the pain. In reality, an easy-to-diagnose mechanical malfunction is responsible for the recurring pain. How I wish the entire medical community would open their eyes and acknowledge the vital importance of the TNS, teeth, muscle, and TMJ! It's easy to see how simple mechanics and physics— —not hormones—cause the pain millions of women suffer from daily. Instead, doctors cite the pain anxiety cycle and blame hormones and women's supposed inability to deal with stress. And why shouldn't they overlook the real, curable cause? The medical and pharmaceutical industries *make hundreds of billions of dollars per year on the backs of suffering women* "treating" them—for years—for issues unrelated to the actual cause of their pain!

SUFFERING FOR SIXTY-FOUR YEARS

The amount of prolonged suffering women endure, not to mention the amount of money they spend trying to survive, is unconscionable. The record in our practice is a woman who suffered migraines for sixty-four years. She was seventy-four years old when she found us. Fourteen years earlier she asked her dentist, a highly qualified dentist by purely dental standards, if the click in her jaw could have anything to do with her migraines. He proceeded to conduct the ridiculous exam the majority of dentists perform: He placed his fingers over her temporal mandibular joints, had her open and close her mouth, and asked, "Does that click bother you?" She said, "No." (It's rarely the click itself that bothers patients with TMJ disorders.) He then sent her out the door to suffer fourteen more years. If the dentist had been required to do a thorough exam, he would have found numerous muscles in spasm and seen that both TMJoints were dislocated, swollen, and inflamed. It wasn't her physician or dentist who referred this patient to our offices, but her granddaughter whom we had treated for severe migraines and vertigo problems. After eliminating the problems her granddaughter and her family feared could be hereditary and would plague her for another sixty years, she sent her grandmother to see me. We were able to get her grandmother off all but one drug this late in the game, and most of her headaches are gone. It wasn't the headaches that were inherited, it was the bite problems that were passed down.

Thumb Sucking Can Cause a Lifetime of Pain

Instead of promoting tooth whitening campaigns, let's start an all-out campaign to stop thumb sucking. This habit not only pushes the upper front teeth forward, it makes the upper palate and dental arch narrower. As a result, children who suck their thumbs are more likely to experience a lifetime of chronic pain because the essential guidance systems won't work the way they were designed to with the narrowed palate and narrow upper arch that thumb sucking often (not always) forces the mouth to develop.

If a football player intercepts one pass and saves the game he is carried off the field in victory. If a campaign to prevent thumb sucking beyond the age of two to two-and-a-half were started, we could intercept millions from lifetimes of pain. This simple, free, preventative solution could especially benefit those in low-income areas where orthodontics are not readily available or affordable.

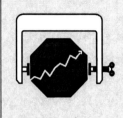

NEWSWORTHY TRUTH

Stress is a trigger that exacerbates pain, but it **is not the cause** of most types of chronic pain and migraines.

This woman is lucky her granddaughter sought help outside the traditional medical system. If the young woman hadn't suffered and found the cure by herself, her grandmother would likely be suffering still. I believe our online survey will prove that, as with this family, most patients are never examined for TNS- and TMJ-related pain, let alone get treated. My prayer is that this book will help make this surgery-free and drug-free cure available to all chronic pain sufferers. To make that desire a reality, women and men who have suffered with this for years must educate fellow sufferers and let them know treatment is available. Then more people would have a chance to seek and find real help.

HOW STRESS CONTRIBUTES TO CHRONIC PAIN

The interferences on the twelve-year molars often produce the unconscious desire to grind and clench the teeth in an effort to grind off these interferences, especially at times of stress. For many people, grinding their teeth or clenching their jaws becomes a nervous habit or stress reaction, which explains why migraine and tension headaches have been blamed on stress for centuries.

I'm not denying that stress plays a role in tension headaches and migraines, but it's a trigger to more clenching and grinding—not the cause of the pain. Here's a simple example: If you have a nightmare, your headache, neck pain, and several other symptoms can reach higher levels because the nightmare intensifies your stress. As we all know, dreams quite often seem far too real. You may even wake in a cold sweat with your heart beating faster. You may also notice that your jaw is sore from clenching or grinding your teeth in response to that nightmare-induced stress. When you place your fingers over your temples and clench your teeth or grind them from side to side, you can feel that huge temporalis muscle in the side of your head. This muscle is also controlled by the TNS; it bulges and contracts right along with the muscle over and over again. When stressed-out, chronic pain sufferers grind or clench their teeth in their sleep, the result is often an excruciating morning headache. Can you see how the tension and pressure could generate a headache and make you feel as though your head has been in a vice all night long?

Sometimes the pain does not wait until morning. For many of these patients, the pain is so excruciating that they have to wake the entire family and drive to the ER. These nights happen far too often for millions of women. As one patient's daughter described it to her mother, "Some of my saddest memories as a child were those nights I was awakened and put in the backseat of the car to go to the ER with the stench of you vomiting into a can in the front seat."

No one disputes that chronic pain leads to increased stress levels, fatigue and depression. The more teeth that are out of alignment, missing, or poorly restored, the more likely that the TN will trigger multiple, chronic pain symptoms. This triggering and re-triggering of the pain cycle can recur for decades. Medical professionals claim they can't figure out what causes migraines and tension headaches to recur on such a frequent basis. This book and the truths within should help you, and the medical profession as a whole, understand the cause for recurring pain. What's more, when you take the self-exam you will see the evidence of it in the wear patterns on the twelve-year molars, the eyeteeth and the upper and lower front teeth.

How we can we allow this pain to continue when there is a solution?

I'm quite sure ninety-five percent of women have never before heard this clear explanation for chronic pain and migraines. I hope these truths help you to understand why this pain has been blamed on puberty, hormones, and stress for so long. It will, hopefully, make even more sense as you read further and take the online survey and self-exam.

How TNS-Related Pain Affects Appearance

I'm probably the only man in the world that looks at the bites of beauty contestants in the Miss America or Miss Universe pageants. These beauties almost all have large, broad, dental arches, which means there is enough room for all their lovely, straight teeth. Not surprisingly, their faces are almost perfectly symmetrical. Symmetry in nature, in art, and in people's appearance is almost universally viewed as beautiful. Proper alignment of teeth, joints, and muscles plays an important part in relation to the development of facial symmetry and beauty. A misaligned bite affects the symmetry of the face, overall head and shoulder posture, and general health as well. TMJ dislocations, imbalanced bites, missing support pillars (teeth) in the skeleton of the skull, and muscle spasms triggered on one side of the face can all lead to asymmetry. When struc-

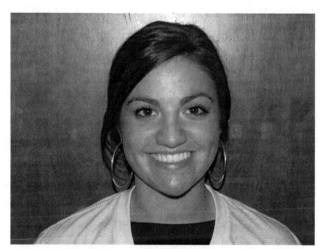

Note the perfect bite and symmetry of this woman's face and posture: eyes equally open, eyebrows and shoulders of equal height, and perfect points on the eye teeth. Such symmetry indicates a perfectly balanced and functioning bite.
Her orthodontist should be proud.

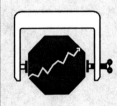

NEWSWORTHY TRUTH

Correcting a person's bite isn't vain or simply cosmetic; it helps that person live a healthier, more active life.

tural support within the bite is inadequate, the patient favors one side more than the other when they chew. This leads to unequal muscular development and facial symmetry. The eye will be open more and the eyebrow higher on the side that the joint is dislocated due to a traumatic blow to the jaw, over-closure of the mouth due to missing teeth, broken teeth, or simply worn down teeth. The side with the greatest loss of vertical height has the least support. The chin may be shifted off midline toward that side, and the corner of the mouth will be higher with a greater wrinkle or crease because of the over-closure and the excess tissue folding over itself. The patient will generally smile on that side the mouth. The level of the shoulders and breasts will also be off balance. These factors all tie into the forward, lateral head posture, which can contribute to scoliosis, slumped shoulders and a dowager's hump, as well as the neck and back pain produced due to weight-shift strains on the joints down the entire body.

Correcting a person's bite isn't vain or simply cosmetic. It helps that person live a healthier, more active life... this is yet another reason why doctors should refer patients to qualified dentists for treatment and that this type of dentistry should be covered by insurance.

One particular patient has been with me since early in my practice before I was treating chronic pain. I first saw her around 1972 when she was just twenty-two years old. At that early age, she already had an abundance of poor dentistry and arthritic TMJoints caused by severe physical and sexual abuse she endured as a very young child.

The Abuse Connection

One reason women are three times as likely to suffer from chronic pain as men is they are more apt to have a history of physical abuse. We have shelters for abused women, but the ongoing pain from a TMJoint dislocated by physical blows may seem inescapable.

One of my patients was sexually and physically abused between the ages of two and sixteen. Her mouth and jaw were damaged as a result, and she suffered with chronic pain and migraines for years. A law passed through our state's legislature required her insurance to cover a portion of her care. But she and her husband still had to cover most of Phase One (the temporary treatment) and the majority of her long-term solutions out of pocket.

Many women remain undiagnosed or untreated due to lack of funds. For these individuals, the physical and emotional effects of abuse can seem endless. Why do they go untreated or undiagnosed? Because these joints and all the other structures supplied by the TNS are still, for the most part, not considered part of the body. Even if the abuse is reported, these areas are rarely examined thoroughly at the emergency room. Months later, when chronic migraines and other symptoms gradually take over their lives, no one examines these women for dislocated TMJoints.

Where can abused women and children turn for relief when no doctor and few dentists are willing to perform a simple exam? And why, when problems are identified by qualified dentists, are the insurance companies permitted to deny these women coverage for a jaw joint dislocated by a punch to the face? Even if the abuse occurs (or occurred) during childhood as it so often does, the necessary repair work is still not covered. As a result, abuse survivors suffer for decades. Unlike cuts and bruises, damaged joints and broken or chipped teeth don't heal on their own. The psychological suffering that comes with abuse is exacerbated when chronic, recurring pain is blamed on the survivor's inability to cope.

At the time, even I was amazed with how much relief we were able to provide for her. After temporary splint therapy was so successful, I was still hesitant to restore whatever needed to be done with crowns until it was more time-tested. So we made her an overlay partial in a harder material than the splint and she did well on that for three or four years. Once we were able to see that the treatment worked for her, we moved on to the permanent solution. Phase Two of treatment included restoring her lower arch of teeth in crowns to increase their vertical height and relieve her arthritic over-compressed joints. She did well with this for about twenty years.

A few years ago this same patient tripped and fell on the slate kitchen floor in her home. Five or six of her upper front teeth broke and her lower jaw was backward into the TMJoint. To repair the damage, she had to have several root canals to save the roots and posts and fusion bridge across the front. We also had to treat her TMJoints all over again. We were successful at eliminating most of the symptoms again. Insurance did cover more for this patient than it does for most patients, but she and her husband still had to pay a good percentage of the cost out of pocket.

PHYSICAL PAIN IS ONLY THE BEGINNING

"I suffered for over four years with daily moderate-to-severe headaches and facial pain. My whole body suffered. My fingers, arms, back, neck, and shoulders all hurt when my head ached. There were countless days I went to work physically and emotionally exhausted. My husband's mantra became 'Susan won't be joining us. She's having one of her headaches.' At The Chronic Pain Solution Center I got my life back. I'm a better wife, a better employee, a better mom, a better everything as a result of this treatment."
—**Susan H., former chronic pain sufferer**

1.

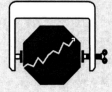

NEWSWORTHY TRUTH

The lack of diagnosis results in many hidden costs in the lives and health of these patients. Here are just a few of the devastating costs of TNS-related pain:

- Years of taking very expensive drugs with numerous, serious side effects that can further harm a person's health,

- Detrimental effects on relationships with one's spouse, friends, parents, children, etc., often occur because these patients are physically and emotionally unavailable when they're in pain,

- Lack of energy, irritability, and absenteeism at work can result in lost jobs and denied promotions,

- Loss of self-esteem occurs when loved ones believe the pain is all in their heads or that they are hypochondriacs,

- Doubt and loss of faith in God in the deepest level of their souls may accompany the bitterness and mood swings resulting from chronic pain.

I believe the loss of internal beauty is the biggest cost of a lifetime of chronic pain. Initially, TN pain creeps into a person's life in small doses. When more severe symptoms develop, it's difficult to remember what may have caused it six months to two years before. Even short-lived pain affects a person's mood and stamina. But loved ones of those who live with severe pain on a daily basis often watch in sadness as that person's entire personality changes. They become moody and irritable and their self-esteem and relationships suffer as a result.

Matters only worsen when patients' family members and friends begin to doubt them, claiming they are exaggerating the pain or are overly sensitive. In a sense, chronic pain sufferers are overly sensitive… but with a real, physiological cause. There are ganglions throughout the branches of the TNS that, once activated over and over from recurring episodes of chronic pain, accelerate or amplify chronic pain sufferers' response to everything from colds, flu, allergies, fatigue, and depression. The good news is: when we eliminate all the stressors on the TNS, these amplifiers quiet down. In turn, the magnified response to colds, allergies, flu and other diseases diminishes as well.

The ex-wife of a physician I treated twenty years ago told me, "I remember people saying to my mother, 'You never smile.' She'd say, 'It hurts to smile.' Now I've got the same thing, and, my ex-husband was always saying to me, 'You never smile.'"

The muscles used to smile, laugh, cry, eat, and cough are the same muscles the TNS triggers into spasm in response to dislocated joints and a poorly supported bite. Smiling, laughing, crying, talking, or eating often increases or triggers more muscle spasms and pain. Most of us have experienced laughing or smiling until our cheeks hurt. It's the same type of occurrence, but for chronic pain sufferers, there is increased pain because these muscles are already over-worked. After her treatment, the physician's wife said, "Wait until my ex-husband hears what was causing all this pain. He was always putting down anything he ever heard about TMJ even though I kept telling him about the muscles in my

---

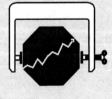

NEWSWORTHY TRUTH

Chronic pain, migraines and tension headaches caused by the TNS and TMJ are *curable*. We know how and why this pain occurs and recurs, and we know how to diagnose and eliminate it in the vast majority of cases without drugs or surgery.

face and the click in my jaw." Had this doctor not been so closed-minded and she had found us sooner, we may have been able to not only end her pain years earlier, but also save her marriage as well.

If saving marriages sounds overly dramatic, believe me, it isn't. In the early years of treating chronic pain, I lived on a small, enclosed cul-de-sac and witnessed firsthand the revitalization of a marriage that occurred when I was able to relieve one of my neighbors of her chronic pain. Suddenly, this mature couple started acting like they were dating again—playing tennis and having fun as a couple and family. Prior to treatment, this woman rarely had the energy or desire to take part in, let alone raise her head, arms and shoulders enough, to play tennis.

The best explanation I've heard regarding the personality change chronic pain sufferers undergo came from a psychiatrist. After hearing me tell him stories of the huge transformations I was witnessing in patients we released from the daily pain that had taken over their lives, he explained, "We are all given a bucket of psychic energy, and we spend it in different ways. Chronic pain patients spend so much of their psychic energy dealing with pain that they rarely have enough left over to reach out and care for those they love and care for the most." In fact, I've noticed that some (certainly not all) of these patients not only lack the energy to love and care for others, but they require so much care and attention themselves that they can suck the psychic energy out of an entire room. Their family and close friends still love and care for them, but even they have limits. Tempers can flare and feelings can get hurt when those limits are tested day in and day out.

At the Chronic Pain Solution Center, we know that at the end of each day we have given someone his or her life back. Most of my patients have suffered for years. My staff and I love knowing that we are not only *freeing them from the prison of pain they've suffered in so long, but also from the malaise of all the prescription drugs they've been taking to mask the pain. They can immediately begin to rekindle broken relationships.* Finally, they are able to become the person, the friend, the spouse, the parent they always wanted to be. Two of my patients said it best. I met the husband of one my patients in a mall and he said, "She's even happy in the morning; I'm not happy in the morning." And one of the moms I treated said, "It's nice for me to have my life back, but it's even nicer for my husband to have his wife back and my kids to have their mom back."

The saddest, and yet most hopeful truth of all is that in most cases, this prolonged suffering and all the collateral damage that ensues as a result are unnecessary. It is time to make the treatment for TNS- and TMJ-related pain available to everyone.

A TIME FOR ACTION

With today's technology and abundance of information, there is no viable reason chronic pain should continue to go undiagnosed, be misdiagnosed, or allow people to suffer. Chronic pain, migraines and tension headaches caused by the TNS and TMJ are curable. We know how and why this pain occurs, and we know how to diagnose and eliminate it in the vast majority of cases without drugs or surgery. But for relief to be widespread, doctors must not be permitted to ignore the cause of chronic pain. People around the globe need to unite and raise the awareness and let the medical and dental world know that ignoring these factors is unacceptable. We must demand that medical insurance companies cover the mouth, the TNS and TMJoints as part of the human body. It is inexcusable to allow insurance companies to deny this treatment claiming it is "experimental," or that this is a dental solution, and therefore not medical issue, while millions, even billions of women suffer. I hope women around the world will agree that this is more than wrong.

Tossing this "political football" back and forth between medical and dental insurance means no one receives coverage—and many cannot afford treatment. This has to be stopped! This is an orthopedic and neurological problem in the head that uses the teeth as vertical support pillars in the skeleton of the head to eliminate the over compression of the TMJoints that are chronically irritating the chief sensory nerve of the head, the TNS.

Women, please stand with me and demand medical insurances cover both Phase 1 and Phase 2 (the long-term cure) of the treatment. You must refuse to accept the practice of keeping patients in pain for profit. Doctors must be required to perform thorough examinations, even with just a ruler or stethoscope, and they must be empowered to refer patients to qualified dentists who can successfully treat the real cause of chronic pain over the dictates of the system that requires they keep people in network or in the clinic.

Can anyone explain 2,500 years of neglect? Can we even comprehend how many billions of people have suffered through the ages, and continue to needlessly suffer today? Hippocrates noticed a connection between crooked teeth and recurring headaches 2,500 years ago. In his Hippocratic oath, which is still sworn to by graduating physicians today, he clearly stated that in the event a physician is unqualified to treat a condition or disease, that doctor is required to call in doctors who know how to treat the problem. The only doctors trained to treat this problem at the cause are dentists. The reality is that if this epidemic of pain afflicted three times as many men as women, it would have been all but eradicated centuries ago. The male-dominated Congress and leaders of governments would have demanded a cure.

Women and their families bear the brunt of this inequity physically, emotionally and financially. I believe that women also hold the power to end this pandemic of pain. Women, united for a cause, are an unstoppable force. If women—if you—get involved and confront doctors and insurance companies, this practice of pain for profit can be stopped.

Imagine living without pain. Imagine your family healthy and whole. Imagine the joy of knowing your daughters and granddaughters won't have to suffer. Now imagine the converse is true... that life continues as it is now. Imagine that doctors are allowed to continue ignoring the proven truths about TNS- and TMJ-related pain. Imagine that your daughters, granddaughters, and great granddaughters are forced to live with chronic pain and migraines because they are denied access to a real cure. **Billions of women are entering dark prisons of hellish pain as you read this today because of this *stoppable* epidemic of pain for profit!** If women unite and make their presence not only heard, but also felt, we could free billions of women from those prisons of pain and from the fear that the debilitating pain will return. They would no longer be labeled hypochondriacs, or told that they're faking it, or that they're weak and simply can't cope with stress. Almost as important as freeing people from the bonds of physical pain is ensuring that everyone has access to treatment and a long-term cure that isn't dependent drugs and surgeries. We must help families escape the financial boondoggle of the pharmaceutical and medical industries.

Like a new "Suff-er-rage movement," I believe this is the time to fight for women's medical rights to be heard and voted on. A scene in the movie *Lincoln* illustrates how adamant men were against women getting the right to vote. The same appears to be true in regard to this women's health issue today. There are more drug lobbyists on Capitol Hill than there are senators and representatives. You can be sure they like the status quo. Women's groups must make their voices and voting presence felt in Washington if this system is going to be changed.

The first suffrage movement started in 1848. *Seventy-two years later* women were finally granted the right to vote in America. But the nineteenth amendment might not have passed had it not been for the countless women who rallied together... and the voice of one woman who used her position of influence: motherhood. In August 1920, Congress was locked in a 48-48 tie over the matter of women's Suffrage. Finally, Harry Burn changed his "nay" vote and broke the tie after reading a letter from his mother, Febb Ensminger Burn, that encouraged him to vote for women's right to vote. Because his mother used her voice, the twenty-four-year-old Freshman Republican Senator switched his vote, and the law passed. The rage of anti-suffragists following that vote, I'm afraid, may be similar to those who would keep the medical system working for profit rather than healing. Burn is rumored to have been chased from chambers and forced to climb out a window where he inched along the ledge of the Capitol until he could escape to safety.

If you think I'm being melodramatic, wait until you read in Chapter Nine about my run-in with an insurance company. This company, despite signed documents from cured patients, wanted to deny their claims and reclaim money they had paid me years earlier. Money is serious business. Those raking billions of dollars—75 percent of which come from suffering women—won't be happy to see the laws and policies changed. Regardless, it's time for things to change.

You Can Make a Difference By Speaking Up!

Here's an example of a story of what must happen to change "the System." Just as this patient did, patients need to go back and ask all their doctors and specialists key questions. You'd be astonished by how much you could help change medical history for chronic pain sufferers today and for generations to come.

This patient, Marie, drove from Atlanta to see me while I was attending a course in Nashville, Tennessee. I had seen a number of websites of Atlanta dentists that said they treated this problem and had the Tekscan computer, but as I was only four hours away from her she decided to drive to meet me in Nashville for a minor exam and evaluation. She had not had a problem with migraines or repeated daily headaches before having had adult orthodontic treatment four years earlier.

After evaluating all structures that could traumatize the TNS in her mouth: her bite, her muscle spasms, and her dislocated TMJoints, I pointed out that only two teeth in her entire mouth made contact when she was chewing or grinding her teeth during sleep: the 12-year molars. Another dentist in Atlanta with a Tekscan computer had told her the same thing: "The orthodontist didn't finish your case very well." I told her to go back with her husband and ask the orthodontist: "Do I have any rights in all of this? I have been suffering for years. It has taken a great toll on my family and our finances. As a result of you not even examining me for this I have gone through years of different doctors, chiropractors, and specialists, and have been prescribed numerous potent and expensive drugs that just masked the pain, but didn't treat the cause. I'm going to have to pay out of pocket for assaults on the chief sensory nerve in my head and face, the TNS, and my dislocated jaw joints, that are causing all this pain. During all these years of suffering I was never even moderately examined by you or your clinic's multiple specialists for these obvious assaults on the TNS that has been known for over a century to cause headaches and migraines. This has had a huge effect on my time with my kids, and my husband has had to pick up my duties numerous times because of my daily pain. I, and my insurance company have paid you and your clinic thousands of dollars over the years while you have just ignored this problem. What are you and your clinic willing to do to help me?"

Within a week of this woman and her husband, the orthodontist wrote her a check for the full amount of her poorly finished orthodontic treatment; and another dentist who misrepresented his use of the Tekscan bite computer in his splint treatment also refunded her $1800.

If thousands of headache sufferers across America and the world, with their spouses, would have the courage to confront doctors, eventually this will reach the administrators of these large clinics and their malpractice insurance providers as well. First, arm yourself with all the truths presented in this book and with how long these truths have been known, and you will definitely catch them ill-equipped to argue with you. End your talk with, "I'd like to hear back from you within a week or I'll have to ask around to find out what rights my family and I have in all of this."

If prisoners of pain and their family members and friends unite, we can change the system that permits doctors not to look for or explain the cause of this curable, life-destroying pain. We can change the system that allows insurance companies to deny effective treatments

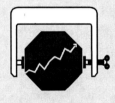

NEWSWORTHY TRUTH

Our mission statement comes from Isaiah 42:7: *To open eyes that are blind* (help the world not only to see this problem, but to be able to examine themselves for this problem if their doctors won't), *to free captives from prison, and to release from the dungeon those who sit in darkness* (free the billions who suffer in prisons of pain).

when they are holding a progress report from the patient stating they are 80 to 90 percent better without drugs. But if we sit on our hands and let the system muzzle our voices, lives and families will continue to be ruined for centuries to come. In that horrible scenario, the system wins. It continues to go unchecked and unaccountable while it brings in hundreds of billions of dollars per year on the backs of women just like you. **We need women and their families to become involved in every state and every country!**

Our mission statement comes from Isaiah 42:7: *To open eyes that are blind* (help the world not only to see this problem, but to be able to examine themselves for this problem if their doctors won't), *to free captives from prison, and to release from the dungeon those who sit in darkness* (free the billions who suffer in prisons of pain). If the women of the world unite and make sure people around the world hear these newsworthy truths, we have a chance at seeing our mission to fruition. I've said before that this information needs to go viral; it needs to become a Facebook, Twitter, email, and YouTube firestorm event. I hope to enlist you in this campaign, not for book sales, but because the medical, insurance, and pharmaceutical dictators are formidable opponents. Just as there are foundations for breast cancer research, heart disease, diabetes, etc., we are going to have to start a foundation for more research and studies related to this relative to its increased frequency with women, elderly and the poor. And also to help with the legal battles that the pharmaceutical and insurance industries are likely to wage against us when this information is made public. Millions of chronic pain sufferers and their supporters must be armed with these truths before we have a prayer of forcing these opponents to listen. Millions of women have already had years of their lives stolen by pain. Many have lost their jobs. Others have lost their families due to the toll of chronic recurring pain. Those costs are too high!

Please! Speak up and be heard. Spread the word about this book, the self-exam, and the online survey. My desire is that these newsworthy truths will spread like wildfire and overtake the Goliaths who were too powerful to defeat before the advent of the Internet. Like toothpaste that is out of the tube, once revealed, the truths about chronic pain will be impossible for the medical, insurance and pharmaceutical industries to hide or deny.

The Truth About the Elderly, Poor, and People in Third-World Countries Who Suffer with Chronic Pain

The elderly and the poor run a close second to women as the most neglected and abused by the medical system when it comes to TNS- and TMJ-related pain. Those in third-world countries fall into a similar category. The reasons for the inadequate care and misdiagnoses these precious people receive are numerous, but the end result is the same. People suffer because they are not properly examined for, or informed about, the true cause of this type of pain.

Patients trust their doctors to help them make informed decisions about their health. In too many cases, however, doctors do not share information about this long-term, drug-free, surgery-free treatment option. And for the poor and those living in third-world countries, healthcare options are limited at best and non-existent at worst. The goal of this book is to educate suffering people and their caregivers about the cause of many types of chronic pain, to empower them with the self-exam, and to offer a potential solution.

Earlier in this book, I explained in detail how this pain starts and why it can continue for decades. I also told you that the teeth need to

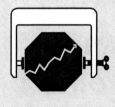

NEWSWORTHY TRUTH

Over time, avoiding one side of the mouth and favoring the other, due to missing teeth, dislocated TMJoints, crooked teeth, sensitive teeth, and broken down teeth, can cause neck strain, shoulder pain, and even lower backaches.

be included in the definition of the skeleton of the skull, and that they must be redefined as essential support pillars in the skeleton. Nowhere is the true function of teeth more evident than in the posture and pain of the elderly and poor. When an individual lacks vertical support due to missing, worn, or broken down teeth, partial or full dentures, or poor alignment, his or her forward and lateral head posture are severely affected. The unnatural posture changes the way a person carries himself. Over time, avoiding one side of the mouth and favoring the other can cause neck strain, shoulder pain, even lower back aches. Unfortunately, most people are completely unaware of how much broken down and misaligned bites contribute to their pain and posture issues.

Most of us in the AARP set come from an era when extractions were the most common and accepted practice for "treating" damaged teeth or crowded bites. Saving teeth wasn't a concern for the dentists or doctors who treated us early in life. Very few of us had orthodontics to straighten our teeth when we were teens; I know of only one girl in my high school who had braces as a teenager. Thankfully, dental care in America has improved significantly through the decades. A sixty- or seventy-year-old person today is likely to have a dentist who attempts to prevent decay and to repair damaged teeth, rather than simply pulling them. If you are like me, you probably have had dental work done as an adult to correct a damaged or misaligned bite. The problem is, not enough dentists have the equipment or training to re-engineer a mouth so that the teeth and jaws find their "happy place." That was certainly true in my case.

I was an inner-city kid from a poor background. My six-year molars were extracted when I was a teenager. As was the way in our neighborhood, these molars were not replaced with bridges. My bite collapsed, (see FIG. 5) giving me a crossbite, as well as TMJ and muscle spasms. My jaw was constantly overstretched. In addition, I inherited enamel hypoplasia: chalky, improperly formed teeth with pitted enamel. Those strikes combined with my poor economic upbringing lead me to learn more about dentistry and TMJ problems.

In dental school, a gifted classmate crowned all but eight of my teeth and placed bridges to close the spaces of the missing six-year molars on the bottom arch. I can never thank him enough for saving my teeth. With my enamel it was my only chance. More than forty years later, I still have all but one of those crowns. Unfortunately, at that time dentists had no idea how to locate the triplane comfort position before building crowns. My bite was crowned into the crossbite that developed when my twelve-year molars drifted into the spaces of my missing six-year molars. The bridges and crowns restored my bite, but they also pushed it back even farther into what at the time was referred to as a centric-relation position. This bite position perpetuated my already existing TMJ problems. Because of the lack of educational resources and technology back in those days, it took several years of trial and error to correct my bite. What I learned during that arduous process helped me become a better dentist.

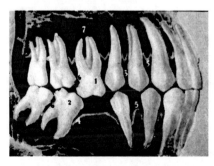
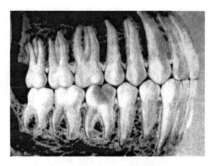

FIG. 5A: A missing molar can cause the bite to collapse.

FIG. 5B: When all the teeth are intact and in alignment, they mesh like gears.

Today, I consider my early dental issues to be a true blessing. They enabled me to see the reality and impact of missing and misaligned teeth in a very practical sense. When I started attending dental courses my personal experience with TMJ issues confirmed the necessity of proper treatment. Even when those in my own profession of dentistry tried to shirk their responsibility in diagnosing and treating TMJ problems, I held true to my course because I understood the pain those joints can cause. The fact that I was able to study these problems from the inside out gave me a supreme advantage. For example, I had read that the TN is proprioceptive, able to detect high spots or interferences at measurements as small as 1/10,000th of a millimeter. When I equilibrated (balanced/measured) my own bite using the Tekscan computer, I was able to understand just how sensitive the TN is and what a whisper of height 1/10,000th millimeter truly is.

I believe my background of poverty gave me the greatest gift anyone could receive: a rewarding career that has allowed me to free many wonderful people from decades of pain and give their lives back to them and their families. My story allows me to speak for the poor and elderly, because missing teeth, crooked teeth, lack of orthodontia, shifted and broken down teeth tell the same story all over the globe. The laws of physics, gravity and the avoidance of pain reflex don't change due to a person's net worth or home country.

In regard to third-world countries, I must admit I have very little experience and data. Few, if any, of these countries do surveys or keep records regarding chronic pain of this nature, and that made it impos-

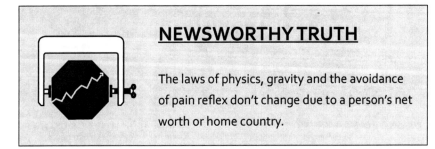

NEWSWORTHY TRUTH

The laws of physics, gravity and the avoidance of pain reflex don't change due to a person's net worth or home country.

sible to get complete data. Remember, most of these people aren't even blessed to be able to read let alone have good dental care. In most of these countries (and even in more advanced countries with socialized medicine), extractions are the most common dental treatment. I've spoken to dentists who have gone on medical missions trips. From what they tell me, their main course of action is to extract painful teeth—not save or restore teeth. Clearly, that only exacerbates the problem. Bites in third-world countries shift out of alignment if teeth are removed from the arch and not replaced, exactly as they do here.

Lack of education and poor or non-existent dental care in third-world countries equates to massive numbers of people suffering worldwide from chronic pain and migraines. Do you see why it is imperative that we all get involved and look for solutions to stop this pandemic of pain? (Don't forget that women comprise 75 percent of these sufferers.) I will tell you this: If this problem is never addressed head on and taken seriously in the United States, the rest of the world is unlikely to devise a solution to help the third-world countries.

THE EFFECTS OF TIME

Teeth have an ideal height that should be maintained, relative to the skeleton and the ideal working length of the muscles with which they chew. Not too high or too low. It's rare in the elderly that their bites are too high. More often their teeth are broken down, missing or tipped over with a crossbite due to missing teeth not being replaced with bridges or partial dentures. When the teeth are broken or worn down, they no longer provide the needed vertical support to prevent over-compression of their dislocated TMJoints. (See FIG. 6.) Just like walking with a stone in your shoe makes you favor one side and avoid the other, a dislocated TMJoint 2 millimeters from the floor of the brain does the same in regard to chewing on one side of the mouth more than the other. When patients favor one side of their mouth for years, they unconsciously develop a forward and lateral head posture.

This forward, lateral head posture causes an abnormal curvature of the spine and is a major issue of poor midline distribution of weight down the body, and a major contributor to multiple types of pain down the body. It's generally followed by rounding of the shoulders causing even more forward distribution of the weight of the upper part of the body. It throws the body off balance, taxing muscles and joints in the neck, back, and shoulders with unnatural strain. Over time, the body's overcompensation for unbalanced weight distribution becomes not only painful, but notably visible. I recently ran into a retired contractor whom I tried to convince years ago that the body is like a building. As a building professional, he would never restore a structure without support beams that were equal on either side, nor would he expect a structure to be sound if it had no beams at all on one side. He understood the analogy, but opted not to listen to me and did not have his teeth—those critical support beams—repaired to their proper vertical

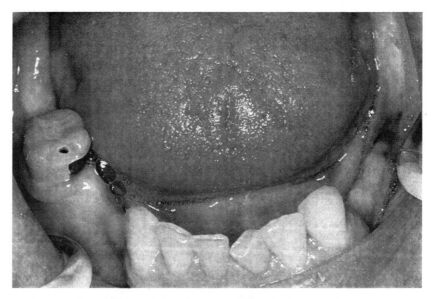

FIG. 6: When teeth are missing, worn down, broken or crooked, they can't provide the necessary vertical support.

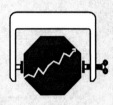

NEWSWORTHY TRUTH

Many dental, TMJ, and even posture issues are correctable even into a person's sixties, seventies, and eighties.

height. Years later, time had taken its toll. His body looked like a capital "C" and the sight screamed constant pain. His head was forward and off to the left and his neck and back curve towards the right and came back toward the left at the hips—and he used a cane to support it all. I guess he figured he needed a beam there for support (the cane). I literally want to cry when I think of how many people like him there are across this globe that are suffering daily, taking drug after drug to kill the pain, and having surgery after surgery that don't address the cause. Gravity and poor posture don't stop just because you operate at the site of the pain. The ingredients for the pain are still there to enable it to return.

In an ideal world, not only dentists, but also all branches of medicine would examine the bite relative to forward head posture. The entire medical community, including dentistry, chiropractors and osteopaths, should look at their patients' bites or dislocated jaw joints as possible causes for chronic pain and migraines. They should offer information about a long-term solution to their patients' forward head posture and the referred pain it causes in the neck, back, shoulder, etc.

Unfortunately, chronic pain sufferers are more likely to be referred "in house" from doctor to doctor and receive little help or hope. For example, an eighty-year-old woman recently came to my clinic for treatment. She was an obvious molar amputee on both sides of her lower arch with no first, second, or third molars on either side. She was in such pain that she had not had a solid meal in two years. Her dentist told her he didn't have a solution and said, "I don't treat this. Maybe you should see your doctor." Her doctor sympathized and said, "I don't treat this, but I can refer you to a neurologist and rheumatologist." But the doctor neglected to add, "They don't treat it either. They just cover it up with stronger and stronger drugs." Sympathizing with my patient, I asked, "Did they refer you to Santa Claus? He doesn't treat it either, but he can make you feel good, too."

Feeling good under the influence of drugs isn't the same as being cured. But the "money tree" doesn't grow as well if you find a solution without the surgeries and pharmaceuticals. Treatment for chronic pain patients often begins with drugs. If the pain doesn't go away, patients are prescribed new drugs and stronger doses. When patients can no longer deal with the pain and side effects of the pills, they often take the next step advised by their doctors: surgery. Rather than giving them a chance to explore a drug-free, surgery-free treatment option—restoring and correcting their bites and addressing TMJ dislocations—doctors ask patients to undergo invasive and permanent surgeries that may or may

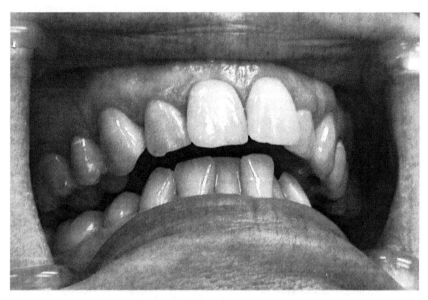

Fig. 7: Before, crooked and crowded teeth caused the jaw to over-compress the TMJoint, leading to assaults on the TNS and daily headaches.

not work. Every day, surgeries are being performed on backs and necks around the world. Unfortunately these surgeries do not address the cause of the weight shift in the penthouse portion of the skyscraper, the vertical support beams (teeth) in the skeleton of the head. Judging by the posture of many of our elderly, how successful do you think these back, neck and hip surgeries are?

THE GOOD NEWS

The amazing fact is that many dental, TMJ, and even posture issues are correctable even into a person's sixties, seventies, and eighties. I've already told you about the woman we treated who had suffered from migraines for sixty-four years.

During my thirty-eight years of dental practice I've treated numerous patients who have lived with chronic pain for thirty or forty years, or longer. We've successfully relieved elderly patients of hearing and vertigo problems. Family members of patients in their seventies and

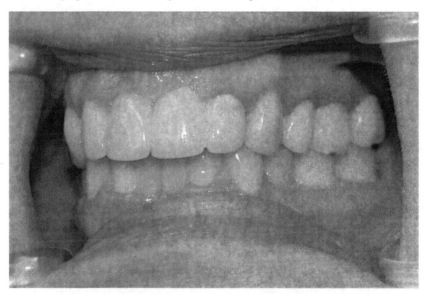

FIG. 7a: After this patient's treatment which included a splint and crowns, the teeth mesh perfectly and provide the essential skeletal support. She no longer suffers from chronic headaches.

eighties watch their loved ones grow taller, stronger, and more energetic as their head posture is corrected and associated neck and pack pain are relieved. You've heard the term, "a new lease on life." That's exactly how many elderly patients feel once they feel whole again and are able to stop taking some of the drugs that kept them in a fog and made them forgetful.

Please understand, I'm not saying prescription drugs don't have a place in our medical care. Certainly, many drugs serve important and necessary functions in modern medicine. Before you start or stop taking any drug, you should talk with your doctor so you fully understand any potential repercussions. That said, we've all heard the fast-talking announcers offer up disclaimers and horrific side effects at the end of drug commercials. Three pages of fine print detailing cautions and potential risks often follow a one-page advertisement for a drug in a magazine. If pain can be relieved without subjecting patients to all those side effects, shouldn't that option be made available to patients?

It stands to reason that increased longevity and quality of life should be included as potential "side effects," or perks that result when the cause of posture problems and pain are addressed. Time and again, I've witnessed patients who, once relieved of their pain, are happier, more energetic, and more active.

ALL PATIENTS DESERVE TO KNOW THEIR OPTIONS

I was on a bike ride in my hometown a couple of months ago when I stopped to talk to an old friend I hadn't seen in a couple of years. I'm convinced it was not by accident that this impromptu conversation occurred just outside an orthopedic and physical therapy clinic. During the forty-five minutes we talked, I saw elderly patient after elderly patient walk in or out the door with forward head postures, walkers, narrow bites, obviously missing teeth, sunken cheeks, and on and on. This scene brought the elderly to the top of the list of those most abused by medicine along with women. Millions (if not billions) live in the dungeons

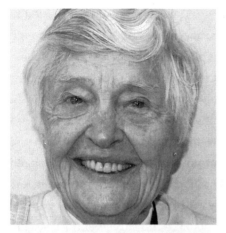

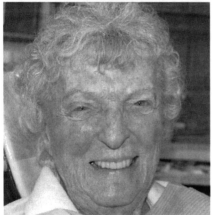

Pat S. (above) will soon celebrate her ninetieth birthday, and Barb M. (below) is in her mid-eighties. Both have great-looking teeth and good facial symmetry.

In 1989 and 1981 respectively, we corrected the vertical height and guidance in their mouths with crowns. Approximately every five years, we spot grind their crowns with the TekScan III bite computer to maintain symmetry and balance.

Neither woman has had plastic surgery, nor do they show creases in the corners of the mouth (other than their smile lines). Both enjoy a full and vibrant life and have avoided pain because of their beautiful, balanced bites.

NEWSWORTHY TRUTH

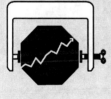

Increased longevity and quality of life also should be included as potential "side effects," or perks that result when the cause of posture problems and pain are addressed. Time and again, I've witnessed patients who, once relieved of their pain, are happier, more energetic, and more active.

of hellish pain because the medical world has been given permission to ignore these vital TMJoints, muscles, and nerves of the head as though they are not part of the body. In effect, these patients are being denied proven and effective treatments that could very well heal them.

While lack of insurance coverage for dental and TMJ issues is a problem, especially for the poor, many of the elderly are able to afford this treatment. They want to know the cause of their pain and are delighted to learn about treatment options that don't keep them drugged up or require them to endure anesthesia and surgery. But their doctors don't bother to explain the very likely cause and solution to their posture problems. When these elderly patients take the survey and self-exam, they will be able to tell if they have a potentially curable condition that has been ignored while they have suffered for years or decades.

At a minimum, chronic pain sufferers—of every age or socio-economic status—deserve to be educated about their options for treatment. They need to be told the truth. They should be given the opportunity to decide if it's worth it financially to explore a treatment that offers

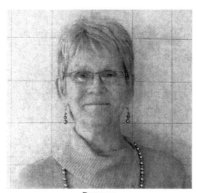

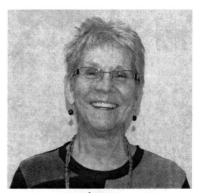

BEFORE **AFTER**

Before treatment, Marge suffered from migraines for 40 years caused by missing teeth and a significantly worn down partial denture. We restored the vertical height to an ideal bite. You can see the improvement the treatment made to her posture—look at the difference in shoulder height in the before and after pictures. I have every confidence that her successful treatment will prevent the need for surgeries on her neck, shoulders, back, and/or hips.

improved health, fewer drugs, more mental acuity, better mental attitude due to less pain, and increased quality of life.

It's Time to Challenge the System

In America, chronic pain transcends economic and cultural boundaries because doctors are allowed not to look for or diagnose the true cause. I know because I've treated many of their patients. It doesn't matter what your social status is, you should at least have the right to know what is causing your pain. **If you have health insurance, the company to which you pay monthly premiums should not have the right to exclude coverage of the chief sensory nerve of the head and face and a joint that is needed to speak, eat, digest, breath, sleep, and for intimacy.**

Patients and their caregivers must confront the physicians, surgeons, chiropractors and dentists to whom they've entrusted their health and well-being. We must make these professionals and the administrators of these large clinics and insurance networks explain why they neglect to examine or refer patients to a qualified dentist to at least explore their options. Proper examination and exploring the right options for each individual patient are essential for healing. Even dentists who specialize in TMJ problems shouldn't rush to permanent treatments or use a one-size-fits all approach. Ideally, patients should first be treated with a splint or orthotic to locate the triplane comfort position of the lower jaw.

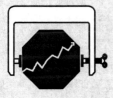

NEWSWORTHY TRUTH

Health insurance companies should not have the right to exclude coverage of the chief sensory nerve of the head and face and a joint that is needed to speak, eat, digest, breath, sleep, and for intimacy.

This determines what height the teeth should be, and where the guidance systems should be placed to position the lower jaw right to left and front to back. The custom, temporary plastic orthotic locates the position that is most comfortable for the TNS, muscles, and joints before moving to Phase Two, the long-term treatment. Phase One allows the dentist and the patient to determine whether or not re-engineering the mouth will work to relieve the pain in the patient's unique and specific case.

Phase Two is the most important advantage dentists have in providing a long-term end to chronic pain and migraines. They can balance the bite using a bite computer to locate high spots and precisely grind them down. Or they can crown or bond teeth to adjust the height of these skeletal supports to reconstruct the bite to the exact triplane comfort position already proven by Phase One to eliminate the pain. Administered properly, this treatment can save individuals thousands (or more) on expensive surgeries and pain medications. More importantly, it allows the elderly to stand tall and lead healthier lives with far less pain.

Unfortunately, as it stands now, if you have private insurance, the orthotic would not be covered at all in twenty-eight of the fifty states, and covered poorly in the other twenty-two. Most insurance policies cover every joint, bone, and muscle in the body, except the jaw joint. For incomprehensible reasons, the jaw joint is not covered by health insurance even if it's dislocated or arthritic and ruining lives with referred pain. Even when dentists can prove that the pain will be eliminated with

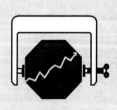

NEWSWORTHY TRUTH

Chronic pain sufferers of every age or socio-economic status deserve to be educated about their options for treatment.

How Great is the Cost of Your (or Your Loved One's) Chronic Pain and Headaches?

Chronic pain can physically, emotionally and financially devastate an individual and his or her family. Take a look at some of the typical monetary costs of TMJ- and TNS-related pain.

It is not uncommon for migraine suffers in America to spend $1,000 monthly for their drug regimen. These drugs include:

- Migraine preventives
- Imitrex, a costly pain medication taken during the migraine
- Antidepressants
- Anti-anxiety medication
- Muscle relaxants
- Sleep enhancers
- OTC pain relievers

In addition, chronic pain and headache patients endure and pay for:

- Repeat appointments with the primary physicians in order to renew the prescriptions for all the meds
- Neurologists
- Rheumatologists
- Ear, Nose and Throat Doctors
- Ophthalmologists
- Physical Therapists
- Chiropractors
- Psychiatrists / Psychologists
- Acupuncturist
- Nutritionists
- MRIs
- CATscans
- Needless surgeries that fail to address the *cause* of the forward head posture and curved spine: sinus, neck, shoulder, lower backs and hips.

the custom triplane orthotic, the money giants see to it that the dentist who is trained to restore the balance permanently is not covered by insurance. As a result, many people have to forgo the treatment, even though they pay medical insurance premiums month after month. No longer can we allow them to toss this back and forth like a hot potato arguing whether this is a dental or medical problem, or whether the treatment is experimental. Meanwhile, patients are denied coverage, and billions across the world suffer daily for decades! **This is a major medical problem, orthopedic and neurological, that can be treated because the skeleton, the teeth, come through the tissue and we can increase the height of these structural support pillars of the skull and eliminate the repeated assaults on the TNS.**

In December 2009, *The New England Journal of Medicine,* a very prestigious journal of medicine, included an article in which the authors stated the teeth and bite should be examined in chronic pain patients. The study found that when these patients were treated with orthotics they received relief in 75 percent of the cases. Unfortunately, researchers also claimed more studies needed to be conducted. **We have centuries of studies that show this connection between these symptoms and the bite!** The medical community and insurance industry should not be allowed to pass this off as experimental.

NEWSWORTHY TRUTH

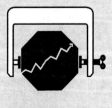

This is a major medical problem—orthopedic and neurological—that can be treated. Because portions of the skeleton (the teeth) penetrate the skin, we can increase the height of these structural support pillars of the skull and eliminate the repeated assaults on the TNS.

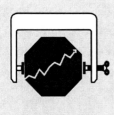

NEWSWORTHY TRUTH

Proper treatment can save individuals (and their insurance companies) **billions** of dollars on surgeries, MRIs, CATscans, endless expensive prescription pain medications, doctor and chiropractic appointments.

Regardless of whether insurance covers an orthotic or alteration and reconstruction of teeth, *does not change the truth.* Ignoring this problem will not make it go away. Enduring surgeries or endless chiropractic appointments that do not address what keeps causing your forward head posture and pain to recur, or keeps masking the pain with expensive prescriptions does not change the truth. John 8:32 says, "The truth will set you free." Ignoring it and pretending your bite is perfect and well supported will not set you free. The cause and the pain will continue to recur until this problem is addressed.

Just as women must organize, so must the elderly. Those of us in our later years must confront doctors, chiropractors, dentists, and pharmacists for not telling us how significantly the mouth and jaw can impact not just dental health and appearance, but a person's overall well-being. I urge you to contact your political representatives on the national and state levels as well to drive change in the insurance industry.

There is strength in numbers and truth, and we have the numbers and the truth that can save individuals billions of dollars on surgeries, MRIs, CATscans, endless expensive prescription pain medications, doctor and chiropractic appointments.[15] It's time to force the medical and insurance companies to make treatment accessible and available to everyone.

Remember, the truth will set you free, but ignoring the truth and not addressing the problem doesn't change the truth or make your pain go away. Take the survey and self-exam and get your friends and loved ones to do the same. If we don't unite and force the medical and insurance industries to take TMJ- and TNS-related pain seriously, nothing will change. There is too much money to be made by simply ignoring or denying the truth.

A Simple Self-Exam
and Survey

Now for the moment you've been awaiting, the **self-exam.** I am honored to offer you this tool as a means of helping you discover whether the TMJoints, your teeth, or other related factors could be the source of chronic pain, either in your life or in a loved one's life. Before taking the self-exam, please complete the online survey at StopTheHeadache.com and skim over the list of symptoms on page 25.

The answers to these self-exam questions are meant to be private. They are to help you determine whether you've ever been thoroughly examined for structural misalignments that would produce repeated assaults on your TNS. Your TMJoint is only one of many possible assaults that may be triggering your recurring chronic pain. Women have been encouraged to perform self-examinations for early detection of cancer to save their lives for years. We need to do the same for chronic pain patients to give them back a quality life, free of pain and the malaise of endless drugs. The world needs to know that all factions of the medical profession have neglected to examine these vital structures that are capable of chronically irritating the TNS. As stated before, the TNS that supplies your teeth, bones, muscles, and joints of the jaw, also covers

Don't Let Ignorance Steal Your Hope

After a severe car accident, a woman who was being treated for a TMJ disorder at another clinic had her orthotic taken away by the clinic's doctor. Soon after, her headaches became so severe that she ended up in the hospital. The resident and the head neurologist both told her she was having a cerebral bleed (stroke) and she would be dead by morning if she left the hospital.

She knew better. She knew she was suffering because her orthotic had been taken away. She left the hospital and found our clinic. Today, fifteen years have passed. This patient's pain and other symptoms have subsided by over 80 percent, and she no longer needs prescription drugs.

In recent years, this woman was diagnosed and treated for cancer. If you have any doubts as to how life-altering the referred pain and symptoms of dislocated TMJoint pain and assaults on the TNS can be, consider this: My patient told me on more than one occasion that she would rather endure her five cancer surgeries, chemo and radiation therapy again than to go back to experiencing the severe headaches, vertigo, sleep loss, chronic fatigue, and depression she lived with on a daily basis before we treated her dislocated TMJoints and assaults on the TNS. This is a very powerful statement to the medical world and to all you chronic pain sufferers.

Help is available! Don't assume the medical profession or their constant expensive testing and drugs are your only hope.

Question: Do you think the doctors in the emergency room that night examined anything listed on the self-exam before telling her she would be dead by morning?

two-thirds of the brain, and the brain-stem down to the third cervical vertebra of the neck. It supplies the eyes, ears, sinuses, tongue, and neck. Amazingly, physicians have been allowed to ignore the TNS.

Before accepting a diagnosis that condemns you to a life of pain—or as in this woman's case, death—take the self-exam to see if it could be your TMJoints or assaults on the TNS that are causing you to suffer.

Trigeminal Nerve System

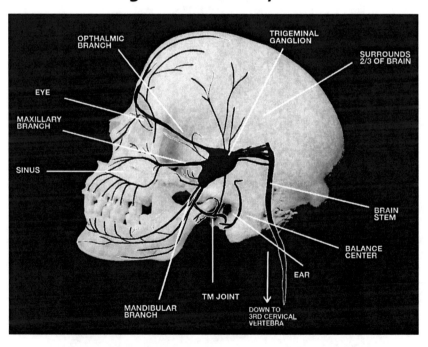

FIG. 8: Refer back to this picture of the
three major branches of the TNS as you take the exam.
Remember: The TNS supplies all the structures mentioned in the exam.

Self-Exam

__Yes __No   Do you hear a clicking, popping or grating sound when you open and close your jaw or while chewing? (See Fig. 9 and Fig. 9a.)

__Yes __No   Does your jaw click or pop when you yawn or open wide?

__Yes __No   Did your jaw click or pop at one time in the past when you opened and closed your jaw?

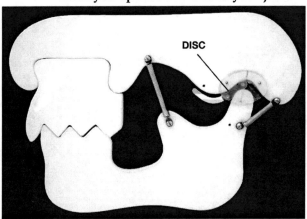

Fig. 9: The disc in the image of the jaw joint acts as a cushion and lubrication between the two bones when it is in the proper position.

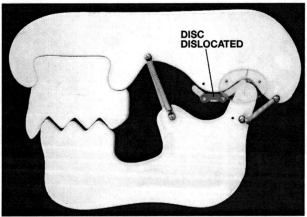

Fig. 9a: In this image, the protective disc of cartilage is dislocated, allowing the two bones to rub against a branch of TNS hundreds of times per day. A clicking sound heard when opening and closing the mouth is the disc popping in and out of a dislocated jaw joint. A grating sound is heard in arthritic jaw joints as these bones rub together.

__Yes __No   Using a millimeter ruler, measure the ability to open your mouth wide from the biting edge of your lower front teeth, to the biting edge of the upper front teeth. Is your opening less than 40 millimeters?

__**Yes** __**No**   **Measure your ability to move the lower jaw right and left. Can you move as far in either direction, or is it harder to move left or right? Measure from the midline between the upper front teeth. Are you able to move 10–13 millimeters right & left?** *(If less when moving left, it means the right joint is dislocated, or vice versa.)*

__Yes __No   **When you swallow do you unconsciously shove your tongue between your teeth?**

__Yes __No   **Do you clench or grind your teeth during sleep or during the day?**

__**Yes** __No   **Do you suffer from chronic neck pain in the morning?**

__Yes __No   Do you suffer from chronic neck pain late in the day?

__Yes __No   Do you suffer from chronic shoulder pain?

__Yes __No   Would your spouse or friends say your head posture is tilted forward or off to one side when you stand and speak to them?

__Yes __No   Do you suffer from neck and back pain?

__Yes __No   Do you suffer from Fibromyalgia?

__Yes __No   Do you have pain in the jaw joints?

__Yes __No   Have you been told that you have a TMJ problem,
                  a click or pop in your jaw joint by your dentist or
                  hygienist?

__Yes __No   Place your fingers above your temple and fan them
                  out along the side of the head while you clench
                  your teeth. You will feel the huge temporalis
                  muscles bulge in the side of your head. Is your
                  headache pain located here? (See FIG. 10.)

__Yes __No   This time clench your teeth together harder for
                  a ten second period and you will feel your neck
                  muscles spasm and tighten up. Do many of your
                  headaches rise from the back of your neck?

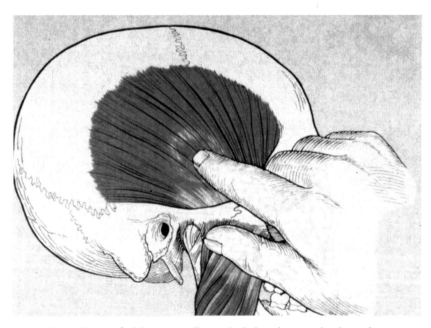

FIG. 10: You can feel the temporalis muscles bulge when you clench your jaw.

__Yes __No   **Have you been in an auto accident and suffered whiplash, struck the dash, windshield or side windows, or received trauma to the jaw in athletics, or from physical abuse?**

__Yes __No   **Do your jaws feel tight or difficult to open?**

__Yes __No   **Is it difficult to keep your jaw open during a simple routine dental appointment?**

__Yes __No   **Are you an "Amputee" in the skeleton of the skull? Do you have any missing teeth that have not been replaced by a bridge or partial denture?** (See Fɪɢ. 6 on p. 102.)

__Yes __No   **Do you have a deep overbite?** (See Fɪɢ. 11.)

__Yes __No   **Do you have an open bite?** (See Fɪɢ. 12 on p. 122.)

__Yes __No   Do you have a deep overjet (lower front teeth do not contact the back of your upper front teeth)? (See Fɪɢ. 13 on p. 122.)

__Yes __No   Do you have a crossbite? (See Fɪɢ. 14 and 14ᴀ on p. 122 and 123.)

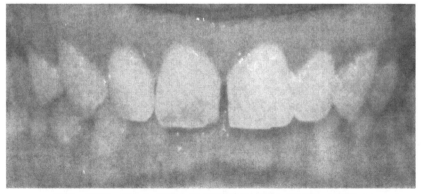

Fɪɢ. 11: With a deep overbite, most of the lower front teeth are hidden when the mouth is closed.

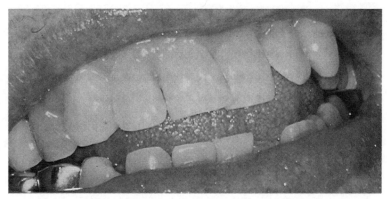

FIG. 12: With an open bite, the upper and lower front teeth are open when the mouth is closed. The needed guidance systems involving the front teeth do not function at all.

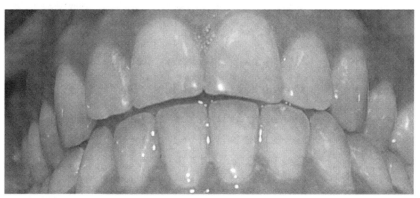

FIG. 13: With an extreme overjet, the lower front teeth do not contact the back of the upper front teeth leading to poor guidance and severe interferences in the molar areas.

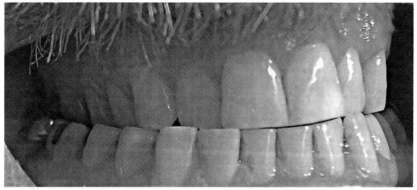

FIG. 14: With a cross bite, the outer cusp tips of the lower teeth line up outside of the cusps of the upper teeth. In a proper bite, the upper teeth should overlap the lower teeth. It can be the poor alignment of the entire arch, one side, or of a single tooth.

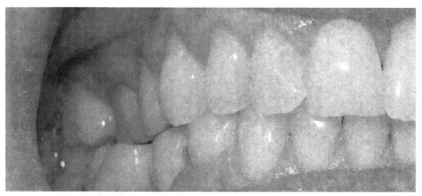

FIG. 14A: With a cross bite, the outer cusp tips of the lower teeth line up outside of the cusps of the upper teeth. This image shows the misalignment of just a few teeth.

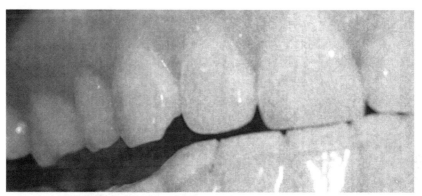

FIG. 15: A worn or flat eye tooth (canine/cuspid) may be the result of grinding teeth during sleep.

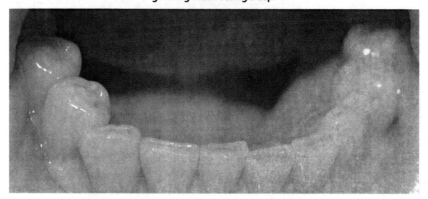

FIG. 16: The biting edge of these teeth are jagged and worn.

__Yes __No   Do you suffer from recurring sharp ear pain, inability to clear ears by swallowing in airplanes or high places, tinnitus (ringing or whooshing in the ears), or hearing loss? (See Fig. 8 on p. 117.)

__Yes __No   Do you suffer from recurring sinus pain, sinusitis, increased mucous production, postnasal drip, and what you believe are recurring allergies with no definite cause? (See Fig. 8 on p. 117.)

__Yes __No   Do you have stabbing eye pain or pressure behind your eyes with your headaches? (See Fig. 8 on p. 117.)

__Yes __No   Do you suffer from teeth that are pressure sensitive when you chew?

__Yes __No   Do you have crooked front teeth?

__Yes __No   Do you have crooked back teeth?

__Yes __No   Do you have very obviously worn/flat areas on the tips of your eye teeth (canines, cuspids)? *(This means you grind far to the right or left during sleep. Try moving the lower jaw to the right and left until the upper and lower eye teeth line up and see if they mesh perfectly. This tells you that you do grind your teeth that far to the sides when you sleep. You would never do that during the day.)* (See Fig. 15 on p. 123.)

__Yes __No   With your teeth together, move your lower jaw to the right and left and check to see if only your eye teeth touch immediately or if your back teeth remain in contact? (See Fig. 4 on p. 78.)

__Yes __No   With your teeth together, move your lower jaw forward and check to see if you immediately touch and ride up on your upper front teeth or if your back teeth remain in contact? (See FIG. 2 on p. 74.)

__Yes __No   Are your lower or upper front teeth worn flat, irregular or jagged on the biting edge as if they are chipping away in small pieces? (See FIG. 16 on p. 123.)

__Yes __No   Have you fractured portions of your back teeth, required root canals or do your back teeth show obvious areas where you have worn them flat? (See FIG. 17.)

__Yes __No   Do you clench or grind your teeth when you are frustrated or under stress?

__Yes __No   Are you aware whether you grind or clench your teeth during sleep?

__Yes __No   Do you suffer from interrupted sleep or inability to sleep?

__Yes __No   Are you awakened by headaches or neck pain during the night or in the morning?

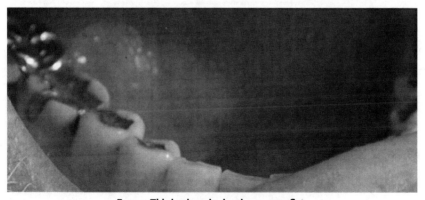

FIG. 17: This back molar has been worn flat.

__Yes __No   **Do you suffer from sleep apnea?**

__Yes __No   Do you snore? Experiment breathing with your lower jaw pulled back and then forward, notice how much easier you breathe when your jaw is forward.

__Yes __No   Do you suffer from chronic fatigue from sleep loss and chronic pain?

__Yes __No   Do you suffer from chronic depression from sleep loss and chronic pain?

__Yes __No   **Do you have full upper or lower dentures, which have back teeth that are worn down or are more than 10 years old?**

__Yes __No   **Do you have upper or lower partial dentures that have back teeth that are worn down or are more than ten years old?**

__Yes __No   **Does your bite feel like you hit only the teeth on one side of the mouth?**

__Yes __No   **If you tap your back teeth together rapidly and lightly does one side feel higher than the other?**

__Yes __No   **Do you have to squeeze your bite together harder to get the other side to hit?**

__Yes __No   In regard to facial symmetry: Do you chew on one side more than the other?

__Yes __No   Is one eye more open than the other?

__Yes __No   Is one eyebrow higher?

__Yes __No   Is one ear higher?

__Yes __No   Is the corner of the mouth higher on one side?

__Yes __No   Do you smile more to one side than the other?

__Yes __No   Are the muscles developed more on one side of your face than the other?

__Yes __No   **If you chew gum (run a test with stiff hard bubble gum) or anything that requires extensive chewing, do you get a headache?**

COUNT YOUR "YES" RESPONSES

If you checked yes to a number of the questions (especially those that are bold,) it's time to get excited. There is a strong possibility that your pain can be eliminated without drugs or surgery.

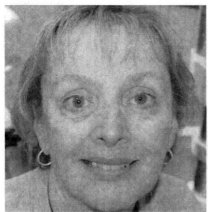

FIG. 17: Facial asymmetry before treatment.   FIG. 17A: Facial symmetry after treatment.

GETTING RELIEF FROM CHRONIC PAIN

Now that you know the likely source of your pain, the next step is getting real help. If you're in, or near, Wisconsin, I would be honored to help you. Contact me at the Chronic Pain Solution Center by phone 414-961-2484 or email help@stoptheheadache.com to schedule a consultation.

Alternatively, contact the American Academy of Craniofacial Pain, aacfp.org or TMJ Equilibration Society at aes-tmj.org for additional resources. Search for a qualified dentist in or near your location whose practice is at least 50 percent dedicated to treatment of TMJ.

Isn't it time you found relief?

Take the Online Survey to
Help Stop Pain for Profit

To change the system that keeps patients in this prison of pain, we need documented proof that this problem is being willfully ignored. Responses to our online survey will help us combat the Goliaths of the medical and pharmaceutical world.

By now, you should realize the obvious connection between your teeth, jaw, TMJoints, and mastication muscles and your pain. *If you read an article that opposes the truths revealed in this book, find out who funded the supporting research. Most such information is funded by pharmaceutical companies. These companies make hundreds of billions of dollars each year while this problem continues to go unrecognized, unexamined, and untreated. The medical industry reaps billions more as well.*

If you haven't already done so, please go take the survey at StopTheHeadache.com. We want to know how many people are seeking help in this arena of chronic pain. You can also connect with me on Twitter at @StopTheHeadache and at Facebook.com/StopTheHeadache. These social media venues will give us multiple methods to contact millions in order to pass legislation to force major insurance companies to cover the TNS and TMJ as parts of the body.

Please: Help us share this vital information.
We need to inform the world before the money giants try to stop this revolution.

WHY THIS TREATMENT WORKS

"I suffered for ten years with daily headaches, excruciating jaw and facial pain. My neurologist told me I had chronic vertigo. The Chronic Pain Solution Center eliminated my pain and vertigo, and I enjoy a far better quality of life with my family. You can too."

—**Laurel B., former chronic pain sufferer**

I HOPE THIS BOOK REFLECTS MY COMPASSION FOR PATIENTS WHO ARE NEEDLESSLY TRAPPED AS PRISONERS OF PAIN. Because you are ambulatory, still walking around, going to work and school, you are viewed as "healthy" on the "wellness line" when the world compares you to cancer, leukemia, AIDS, or diabetes patients. Just as there are tests for other diseases, there are tests and diagnostic signs for these chronic pain symptoms. The problem is, doctors don't conduct the tests or check the diagnostic signs. Because chronic pain prisoners go unexamined and diagnosed, no one believes their pain is real. This lack of support makes chronic pain more difficult to deal with than other diseases over time. Even the people who love these patients must begin to doubt them and start to believe the doctors who say, "It's all in their head," or, "They can't cope." Unfortunately these same doctors who have stethoscopes around their necks, are **permitted not to use them** to examine the TMJoints for dislocation and traumatic assaults on the TNS.

THE BASIS FOR TREATMENT

In *The New England Journal of Medicine,* one of the most prestigious medical journals in America, a December 18, 2008 article titled "Temporomandibular Disorders" outlines why the medical profession needs to give more attention to the teeth, bites, and TMJoint problems. This article supports many of the points I make it this book. Its coauthors, Steven J. Scrivani, D.D.S., D.Med.Sc.; David A. Keith, B.D.S., D.M.D.; and Leonard B. Kaban, D.M.D., M.D., offer the following facts:

- Ear pain, stuffiness, tinnitus, dizziness, neck pain and headache are commonly related symptoms of temporomandibular disorders.

- In some patients, a chronic temporomandibular disorder develops with persistent pain accompanied by physical, behavioral, psychological and psychosocial symptoms similar to those of patients with chronic pain syndromes in other areas of the body (e.g., arthritis, lower back pain, chronic headache, fibromyalgia, and chronic regional pain syndrome.

- TMJoint disorders often accompany coexisting psychopathology (anxiety and depression disorders, post-traumatic stress disorder, and childhood physical, sexual, and psychological abuse).

- Symptoms are often worse in the morning for patients who clench or grind their teeth during sleep.

The authors recommend that a physician's physical exam include observation and measurement of mandibular motion (maximal interincisal opening, lateral movements and protrusion, palpation of the muscles of mastication (masseter, temporalis, medial and later pterygoid muscles), the cervical musculature (palpation of the anterior and posterior neck), palpation and auscultation (stethoscope) on the TMJoints, and examination of the oral cavity, the teeth, and occlusion. They also note that noise in the TMJ on mandibular movement is frequently present in patients with TMJoint disorder. However, noise alone is also a very common finding among people who are completely asymptomatic. I **have no argument with this truth. I do pose the major argument that all patients who experience noise in their TMJoints and suffer daily should be examined and referred to well-trained dentists for treatment, rather than be prescribed drugs for the pain.**

The article even points out that appropriate therapies such as custom-made hard acrylic orthotics are successful in alleviating the pain symptoms of TMJoint dysfunction in 70 to 90 percent of patients. The authors explain that as a general principle, tooth-to-tooth interferences and discrepancies in the anterior posterior jaw position (a bad bite) should be eliminated and missing teeth replaced in an effort to achieve optimal dental occlusion and chewing function.

They further state that the patient's dentist ought to be able to construct the appliance needed. At this point, I have to disagree with them, because the average dentist has not been trained adequately in the design and development of multiple splint options, including guidance systems and moving the lower jaw forward. This is a very involved area of dentistry, and a patient should not just be referred to their dentist who rarely treats this or just dabbles in it. The sad outcome for patients whose dentists don't specialize in this treatment is that they not only remain in pain, but, worse than that, they now think they have been treated for this problem and rule it out of their future treatment options. The result is a lifetime condemned to pain, when really, the problem wasn't the diagnosis. It was the fact that they weren't treated by someone with specialized equipment and training in this area of dentistry.

That one point aside, I'm thankful that a prestigious publication like *The New England Journal of Medicine* took note of this issue and gave it some much-deserved attention. Treatments that include custom-made orthotics need more recognition because of the significant relief they can offer—without the need for surgery or prescriptions.

ALTERING THE SKELETON WITHOUT SURGERY

In Chapter Two, "The Anatomy of Chronic Pain," we identified some of the unique points that make dentistry the obvious and ideal solution to relieving patients of TNS- and TMJ-related pain. Most notable is the fact that the teeth are the only place in the human body where the skeleton comes through the skin. (See Fig. 18.) This important truth explains why balancing the bite and providing adequate support and guidance for the jaw can offer a permanent cure for this hellish pain of recurring headaches, migraines, neck pain, and the symptoms listed

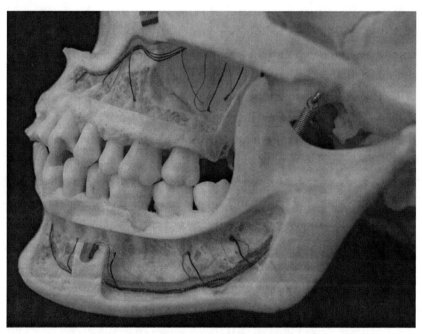

FIG. 18: The teeth are the only place in the human body where the skeleton comes through the skin.

earlier without surgery. It explains why this life-altering pain recurs for decades if nothing is done to address the cause.

The teeth are the vertical support pillars of the skeleton of the skull that not only stop your jaw from over closing, but also guide your bite into the proper position relative to midline. When your teeth are out of alignment, they misguide your bite and create a strained position off midline. If you are missing teeth, especially vertical support pillars in the back of the mouth (the molars), you are an "amputee of the skeleton of the skull." With nothing there to stop your jaw from over closing on that side, the entire bite system (occlusion) is pushed severely out of balance, triggering a series of events that result in a host of painful symptoms.

The fact that the skeleton is exposed through the skin works to our advantage in devising a solution. Because the teeth are exposed, we can alter them without surgery. The effect is that stresses on the muscles, bones, joints that are repeatedly irritating the TNS are eliminated. When that happens, the pain is also eliminated. Dentists who are trained in the fine points of occlusion (bite) can permanently change the skeleton without surgery.

Perhaps the greatest benefit of orthotic treatment for TNS- and TMJ-related pain is that we can eliminate 80 percent of the pain before proceeding with any permanent changes to the teeth. To my knowledge, no surgery can promise a known result beforehand. You have the surgery first, and are then told, "I'm sorry it didn't have the positive effect on your sinus, neck, or back pain that we thought it would." In contrast, at our office, you are not offered Phase Two treatment, the permanent alteration of the teeth and bite, unless you have improved and your pain has decreased by 80 percent or more. Please, before you allow a surgeon to operate to relieve any of the chronic pain symptoms outlined in this book, do the self-exam in Chapter Five. See a qualified dentist for a more thorough exam, and, at a minimum, see if Phase One of the treatment helps relieve your pain.

In Phase One, a custom, computer-balanced, hard mandibular orthotic made of acrylic is used to temporarily provide the patient with a perfect bite in plastic and provide ideal guidance that will enable us to find that triplane comfort position, the Happy Place discussed in Chapter Two. Using the sensitive Tekscan bite computer, Shimstock 5/1000ths of a millimeter thick metal foil, and red and blue articulating paper (that is what all other dentists use), it is possible to locate the precise triplane comfort position of the bite where the entire trigeminal nerve system is relieved of most chronic irritations. By locating the position that the lower jaw wants to be in relative to the sagittal plane (right to left), frontal plane (front to back) and horizontal plane (vertical height of the teeth), we find the position where the pain is gone or reduced by 80 percent or more: the Happy Place.

Even in the event that the TMJoints are dislocated and are rubbing bone on bone against a branch of the TN, we are able to use the same type of triplane orthotic to prove that we can eliminate the chronic pain without drugs before permanently making changes to the teeth themselves. Since we have access to the skeleton without cutting the patient open, we can engineer the bite to that position (again using the Tekscan bite computer to balance the bite). We do this by increasing the vertical height of the teeth by crowning certain teeth or designing a harder version of the plastic orthotic, an overlay partial, that won't wear down like the plastic. If you are missing teeth throughout your mouth, you will need a prosthesis to replace the amputated teeth that are not there to stop you from over closing. Thus we can change the skeleton permanently, thereby relieving or eliminating most of the assaults on the TNS thereby preventing the pain from recurring.

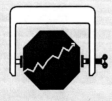

NEWSWORTHY TRUTH

One of the greatest benefits of orthotic treatment for TNS- and TMJ-related pain is that we can eliminate 80% of the pain *before* proceeding with any permanent changes to the teeth.

Avoiding Unnecessary Neck Surgeries

Two patients scheduled for neck surgery for bulging discs between C5 and C6 ran into one of our patients and put a hold on their surgeries after hearing about the treatment and relief she found in our practice.

One was a molar amputee. No one had looked into her mouth or mentioned anything about missing teeth being a possible cause of her poor head and neck posture. The other patient was a male. Both his wife and his neurosurgeon called our office saying there was no way his dislocated jaw had anything to do with his bulging disc.

Both patients received treatment in our office—treatment that addressed the physical cause of their neck problems. Twenty years later, neither of these patients has needed neck surgery.

Medical insurance would have paid many thousands of dollars for both neck surgeries, but paid little or nothing toward the orthotic and Phase Two treatments these patients needed to increase the vertical skeletal support in the skeleton of the head. The treatment corrected the head and neck posture on a long-term basis and saved them from having to undergo painful surgeries.

Don't let doctors tell you that because you have a bulging disc, a deteriorating disc, cervical degeneration or arthritis of the spine that this treatment won't work. Degeneration and spurs on the vertebrae occur when your head is off to one side and the neck muscles tighten on one side more than the other. Consider how a tight string on a bow and arrow forces the wood to curve. When the muscles on one side of your neck are tighter than the other, it creates a pull. Only the bow in this case is your spinal column that is only a series of building blocks attached by muscles and ligaments. Over time, the bones on the inside of the curve between the vertebrae will wear more and form a spur (cervical degeneration or arthritis).

If a prosthesis is used to replace missing teeth, the head posture corrects itself. As the muscles in the neck relax, they stop over compressing the vertebrae and the pain subsides.

People all over the world are having atrocities done to them — metal rods put in their back or neck or fusion of vertebrae in the neck or back — without doctors or dentists ever looking in the mouth to see if imbalances or missing teeth are causing the forward head posture and rounded shoulders that apply excessive pressure on the muscles and discs of the neck and back. Again the medical community is permitted to ignore the mouth, the teeth, the muscles, bones, and joints that are all supplied by the TNS, which also supplies the eyes, the ears, sinuses, throat, the neck, and surrounds the brain and receives 50 percent of the sensory input going to the brain. How do they get to ignore assaults on a nerve of this importance?

Another unique attribute of the TNS is that it is proprioceptive to a tolerance of 1/10,000th of a millimeter. Not all patients are so sensitive to interferences, but as we refine the treatment in Phase Two, we find that some chronic pain patients are definitely this sensitive. Filing the tooth or the crown ever so slightly can provide substantial relief. Some of my patients try to explain to their coworkers or friends just how small the adjustment is and how amazingly it reduces their symptoms, but no one understands. One-ten-thousandth of a millimeter, is such a small amount, and yet the bite computer's technology and Shimstock allows us to see precisely where a tooth needs to be adjusted to eliminate interferences and pain.

Since the teeth are exposed and out in the open, we can lengthen, shorten, move around or reshape them as needed. When we improve the balance and guidance systems of the TNS, the pain doesn't return. In contrast, patients who see a massage therapist for example, may experience relief for a few days; but because only the muscles are realigned and the skeletal imbalances in the bite are left unchanged, the pain eventually returns.

The next section goes into a little more detail about the actual process we use at the Chronic Pain Solution Center. It will help you understand exactly how we alter the skeleton without surgery.

EXAM AND TREATMENT PROCESS

I highly recommend that a spouse or loved one come with you for your first appointment. It will do you, the patient, a world of good to have your closest caregiver finally hear from a doctor that your pain is not "all in your head," even though these structures are all in your head. The source of your pain will be so obvious by the end of your first appointment that you both will be wondering why no other doctor has ever examined you for this problem.

Much of what we do in the first appointment is covered in the survey and self-examination portion that hopefully you have already taken. It will give you a much better understanding.

Before conducting the examination, we take a complete health history and find out how many of the symptoms you suffer with and at what age your symptoms started relative to puberty and the eruption of your twelve-year molars and your canines. We'll find out how many years you've been suffering. You'll be asked to list the prescription drugs you're on at present, as well as the drugs you've taken in the past to deal with this pain. We'll also trace back through the years to determine when the problems started. Common questions during this section include:

- Have you been in any car accidents?
- Have you ever had a blow to the head?
- Did you ever fall off a bike and hit your face or head?
- Have you ever fallen on your face?
- Have you ever been battered, or physically or sexually assaulted?
- Do you remember any blows to the face or head during sporting accidents?
- Do you recall when your jaw started clicking and what may have caused it?

After taking a thorough history, we'll take you into another room where we will examine your mouth, TMJoints, teeth, muscles of mastication, head, neck, shoulders, and back. You'll see how easy it is to examine for this. We'll simply look in your mouth to find wear patterns in your teeth and use the Tekscan bite computer to diagnose how quickly your guidance systems engage. Then we'll use a stethoscope to listen to your TMJoints to hear whether or not they're clicking, which indicates if your jaw is dislocated, and note if you have a grating sound (crepitus) which indicates if the bones in the joint are rubbing bone on bone and you have either arthritis or a perforated disc. Then we will use a millimeter ruler to measure the maximum opening of your jaw, and how far you can move the jaw right, left, as well as forward, noting at the same time whether your jaw deviates to one side or the other, as you open wide or move forward. In other words we record much of the same information as we've included in the self-examination.

Then, using my index finger, I palpate the muscles in the temple region and other muscles that are involved in chewing and clenching your teeth. These are some of the most powerful muscles in the body. These muscles, combined with the TNS, run your entire gnathological system, the mechanical network of the chewing machine at the base of the skeleton of the skull that connects to your neck as well. If this system is out of alignment or functioning improperly, it will cause certain muscles to go into spasm.

Note that I said the system is out of alignment; this is an orthopedic (muscle, bones, and joints) and neuromuscular problem. It isn't only about your teeth. The teeth are just static support pillars, but they can be used to eliminate stresses and torque on the entire neuromuscular orthopedic system of the head and neck. Major medical insurance companies like to argue with this truth. Often, they deny treatment, claiming your pain is a dental or TMJoint problem, neither of which do they cover. However, the truth is your pain is a major medical issue. It's absolutely ludicrous that major medical insurance does not have to cover a system that is so vital to a person's very existence when you pay thousands of dollars in medical premiums to cover every joint in your body—not all but one; and to cover every nerve—not all except for the largest of the twelve cranial nerves that surrounds the brain.

Palpating muscles is not rocket science. During the examination when we apply pressure to the muscles of mastication (chewing muscles), your neck, shoulder and back muscles, we have you grade them on a scale of zero to five. Zero doesn't hurt at all, one is tender, two is uncomfortable, three actually reaches the level of pain, four hurts so bad you don't want me to do that again, and a grade of five is so severe "if you do that again I'll kill you." There's no mistaking the fours and fives. They're very obvious, and it ties together the connection to areas of your pain in many instances. The exam allows both you and your spouse to realize the connection between your symptoms and physical state. Many patients break down in tears feeling they have finally found the cause. They are able to connect the dots; it all makes sense. Using these basic examination techniques, we will be able to give you a good idea if the cause of your pain is related to your TMJoints and TNS.

The next part of the exam uses a high-tech bite computer. For the first time in your life, you'll be able to see the imbalances and lack of support or guidance in the mouth and skeleton of the skull. All of these bite issues can irritate the TNS and cause both local and referred pain. You'll be able to see on the computer screen for yourself how well your teeth align and how quickly your guidance systems engage. (See FIG. 19 and 19A on p. 142.) You probably knew that spacecraft and airplanes have guidance systems, but not your mouth. In your mouth, these guidance systems are supposed to keep your jaw in proper position. Now we have technology that enables us to observe whether your eyeteeth are providing the necessary lift off from your twelve-year molars as thoroughly and quickly as they should. This is key to eliminating your pain! We will also use an electromyograph (EMG) to measure muscular activity and listen to TMJoints via sonar or vibration analysis—much more sensitive than my ears and a stethoscope—while at the same time tracking your jaws as you open and close. This technology gives us valuable information that proves why the problem exists and how best to address it.

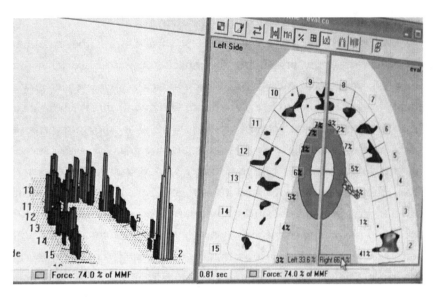

FIG. 19

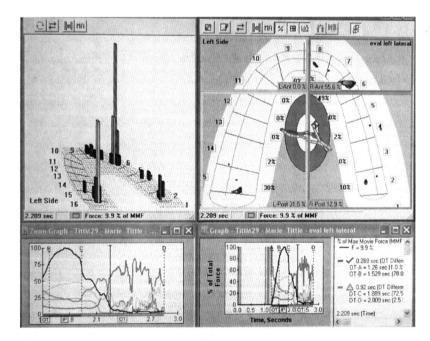

FIG. 19A

At the Chronic Pain Solution Center, we pride ourselves on educating our patients and spending time to help them understand what has been going on and why their problem is so treatable. For example, using pictures we can explain how extensive the TNS is. We also demonstrate how the TMJoints rotate on a vertical as well as a horizontal axes as they translate at the base of the skull out of the fossa with or without the disc in place. This knowledge will give you a new understanding of your pain. We encourage our patients to ask as many questions as they like.

Once all the exam data is gathered we can explain your case with information specific to your test results and give you an estimate of the cost for Phase One.

PHASE ONE

Treatment begins by taking impressions of your upper and lower arches. We then have a plastic MARA (mandibular anterior repositioning appliance), a lower orthotic or splint, custom made for you. The splint allows us to relieve the multiple assaults on the trigeminal nerve system by decompressing the TMJoints and removing trauma caused

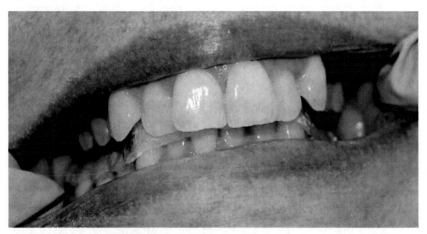

FIG. 20: A splint is made of clear plastic, fits over the lower teeth and is difficult to see. It's a custom fit removable orthotic that enables us to locate the triplane comfort position (Happy Place) of the mandible, muscles and both jaw joints all controlled by the TNS.

Skip Dangerous Treatments and Look Better!

Many migraine sufferers pay for injections of Botox, a derivative of the most deadly toxin on the planet, to deaden the branches of the TNS supplying the muscle in the temple, the temporalis muscle. Each treatment costs $2,000 to $3,000 and lasts only three months. Meanwhile, the person looks like a mannequin because the muscles are basically paralyzed by the Botox. This deadly toxin is injected above and around the eyes. What are the drug companies going to say ten years from now? "I didn't know that it would affect your eyesight."

In contrast to Botox, this treatment addresses and treats the cause of the migraine and provides a long-term cure that keeps the facial muscles fully functional. It's like a facelift from the inside of the mouth. The increased vertical height of the teeth relaxes the muscles, restores facial symmetry, and fills out some of the excess skin causing wrinkles, especially in the corners of the mouth. You won't just feel better; people will ask what you had done.

by crooked and missing teeth from the equation. Designing and using specific guidance systems with the bite computer, we use this clear plastic MARA to find your triplane comfort position—the position one of my patients named the "Happy Place." (See the illustration on p. 50.) Using this technology, we are able to give you a perfect bite in plastic and prove to you that we can eliminate your pain before recommending the long-term treatment solution in Phase Two.

Once your pain subsides by 80 percent or more, the goal is to maintain that "happy place" for one-and-a-half to two months. We want to confirm that we have found your unique solution. This waiting period is used to prove the effectiveness of the treatment. As we get closer and closer to the "happy place" the number of necessary adjustments decreases because you won't clench or grind nearly as much as you did when you started treatment.

When we're both convinced Phase One treatment has worked, it's time for us to gather the information we've learned from the mouth models mounted in the triplane comfort position. By analyzing these models, we are able to accurately identify your ideal jaw position. From this information, we determine what we need to do to recreate and stabilize the bite, lower jaw, both joints, and TNS to that spot for a long-term final solution or cure. People who don't achieve at least 80 percent relief are not offered the Phase Two, long-term cure option. Unless, or until both the patient and I are very confident of the outcome, we do not move to the long-term treatment phase.

PHASE TWO OPTIONS

Until we actually find that triplane comfort position or "happy place," we have no idea what Phase Two will entail. Once we have that information, though, we are able to make the move from a temporary treatment to a long-term solution that eliminates or greatly reduces chronic pain, tension headaches, and migraines—without surgery or medication.

The least invasive and simplest cases involve computerized balancing of the bite using the Tekscan computer. By filing down or building up even a few teeth it may be possible to eliminate your pain. Imagine if this is all you really needed and you would have spent your entire lifetime in pain because your dentist didn't check you out on the Tekscan bite computer.

Sometimes Phase Two requires crowning certain teeth along with an equilibration. It could be that only the guidance teeth need to be crowned to enhance guidance along with the equilibration. Sometimes it's the right side or the left side that needs to be built up or the entire lower arch needs to be built up with crowns, but it's important and exciting to remember this: You live in a time when technology enables

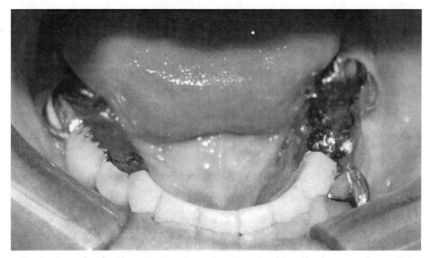

FIG. 21: An option for Phase Two treatment is using a durable orthotic, an overlay partial covered with titanium metal in areas of most stress, and tooth-colored acrylic in areas of lower stress. This maintains the long-term support for the jaw in the high stress areas and eliminates assaults on the TNS *without surgery*.

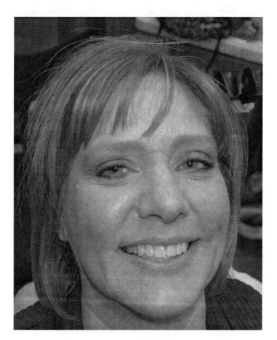

When the lips are relaxed, the overlay partial
is not noticeable.

you to have this done and provide a long-term cure for your pain. Do you realize how many generations in past centuries never had this option?

In the event that the entire lower arch is involved, we have a lesser expensive method which is making a durable orthotic, an overlay partial covered with titanium metal in high stress areas, and tooth colored acrylic in low stress areas. This is strong enough to withstand the hundreds of pounds per square inch of bite pressure without wearing down like the plastic orthotic. (See Fig. 21 on p. 146.)

Another option that is offered by some is orthodontics. I've used it in minor cases. I have reservations as to whether orthodontics can be as accurate at reproducing the triplane comfort position for the long-term cure. Having said that, I am certainly willing to learn from specialists who are educated in the fields of both chronic pain relief and orthodontics. Perhaps we could find yet another viable treatment option. During the growth and development years of young children and adolescents it is very definitely a viable option, but the orthodontist must keep the alignment of the joints as well as the teeth in mind while moving the teeth and expanding the arches to ensure the teeth are retained in that position and will not move back out of alignment. With crowns and overly partials this is not a problem because the teeth were not moved.

People whose bite discrepancies, dislocations, and muscle spasms involving the TNS are less severe may be able to wear orthotics only at night while going without it comfortably during the day. In these cases, the orthotic will need to be surfaced one to three times per year to maintain the perfect bite.

Again, the only way to determine which Phase Two treatment is the best option for your unique situation is to study the bite after Phase One therapy is complete to determine how much of a discrepancy exists.

DON'T IGNORE THE TRUTHS

All chronic pain sufferers should be very excited to find out that this is a very treatable problem. It's orthopedic and neurologic in nature, but it is basically a structural engineering problem in the skeleton of the skull involving guidance systems and vertical support columns like any building, and it's very treatable. Please don't let anyone tell you otherwise until you have seen a specialist whose practice is at least 50 percent dedicated to this treatment. Our practice has been 80 to 90 percent dedicated to this treatment for over 30 years. You do not want someone who just dabbles in this. You need to talk to somebody who's going to show you the intricacies and how much common sense the treatment makes.

As I've said throughout this book, the solution for chronic pain will come when doctors, dentists, insurance agencies, and patients stop ignoring the truths about these critical structures. Yes, even patients ignore these truths by neglecting to seek out and obtain relief simply because their insurance refuses to cover the treatment. Ignoring the truth about the cause of your pain doesn't change the truth. You will still be suffering next year unless you believe these truths and make it a clear priority for you and your family to pay for this treatment. When this pain is gone, it is like a miracle; it will change your whole world.

If you haven't already, take the self-exam provided in this book, as well as the survey at StopTheHeadache.com. Don't allow this pain to steal your life any longer. By reading this book, you have taken the first step of educating yourself about the options. Now take the next step and get help.

NEWSWORTHY TRUTH

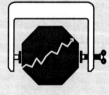

Ignoring the truth about the cause of your pain doesn't change the truth. You will still be suffering next year unless you make it a priority to get proper treatment. When this pain is gone, it is like a miracle; it will change your whole world.

PART II

PAIN FOR PROFIT

FOLLOW THE MONEY

For three years I desperately sought relief through repeated X-rays, heat packs, cold packs, message, ultrasound, TENS units, electrical stimulation, satellite ganglion blocks, trigger pain injections, nerve testing, blood work, MRIs, pain medication, muscle relaxers, anti-inflammatory medications, migraine headache medication and narcotics, anti-depressants from multiple doctors, dentists, physical therapists, chiropractor, neurologists, oral surgeons and internists.

Unfortunately, all the suffering and medical expense resulted in the loss of my job, my income, my ability to drive a car and clean my own house. My career was ruined and a tremendous strain was put on my relationship with my husband and family.

I was declared disabled by my family doctor. I also developed an ulcer from the continued high dose of anti-inflammatory pain medications.

In April, I began splint therapy with Dr. Richard Seymour. It was my salvation! By July, I had improved enough to drive myself to doctor's appointments and was starting to get through each day with less medication. By January, with an 80 percent improvement, I was taken off disability.

—Deborah, chronic pain survivor

Follow-up note from Dr. Seymour: Think of the money saved by the insurance and government when Deb got off disability. She now has two children and has started her own business.

IN SECTION ONE, WE EXAMINED THE CAUSE OF CHRONIC PAIN. You learned why women are more susceptible to this type of pain. You learned that trained dentists can alleviate chronic pain using drug- and surgery-free treatments. I also explained that the entire medical community has been permitted to ignore the TNS, TMJ and these proven and effective treatments. In Section Two, we are going to take a look at why doctors are not required to tell patients they have some of the obvious signs of pain associated with TNS and TMJ pain, nor required to tell them that a treatment exists.

IS THE "IN-HOUSE" OR "NETWORK" SYSTEM KEEPING YOUR IN PAIN?

Have you ever suspected that your doctor or the administrators of your health plan are keeping you in pain? In essence, that may not be too far from the truth. In the United States, many doctors, clinics, hospitals, and insurance companies operate under an "In-House" system of health care. The system is a huge part of the problem.

I'm sure you are aware of how this system works. First, you must go to a general practice doctor. He or she may prescribe medicine for your pain. When drugs don't do the job, the doctor will refer you to a specialist within your "network." The specialist will prescribe different drugs, expensive tests and/or invasive surgeries. When those "treatments" don't work, the specialist may refer you to yet another doctor or to a physical therapist within the network. Not once does one of these professionals examine your mouth or jaw, as you will clearly see when you take the online survey.

Once in a great while, a caring doctor, nurse or physical therapist may examine a patient's the mouth and jaw, see the signs of TNS-related pain and recommend that the patient seek treatment outside the network. If this happens once, it is unlikely to happen again. Why? Physicians are encouraged not to refer patients (a.k.a. the money tree) out of their network—even when no treatment for the problem is available "in house" or even if more effective treatments could be received elsewhere. In fact, administrators put pressure on medical professionals not to refer patients to someone outside the network.

The responsibility of all healthcare professionals is to make sure patients receive the best possible care. To that end, the Hippocratic oath states that physicians will call in other doctors if the patient's condition is beyond the scope of their training. It does not say for dentists or physi-

Excerpts from the Modern Version of the Hippocratic Oath

I swear to fulfill to the best of my ability and judgment, this covenant:

I will not be ashamed to say I know not, nor will I fail to call in my colleagues when the skills of another are needed for a patient's recovery.

I will remember that there is art to medicine as well as science, and that warmth, sympathy, and understanding may outweigh the surgeon's knife or the chemist's drug.

I will apply, for the benefit of the sick, all measures that are required, avoiding those twin traps of over treatment and therapeutic nihilism (the belief that there is no objective basis for the truth).

I will respect the hard-won scientific gains of those physicians in whose steps I walk, and gladly share such knowledge as is mine with those who are to follow.

cians, "We will keep all patients 'in house' when we don't have anyone in our clinic that handles this life-stealing suffering." Medical physicians really can't treat the cause; they can only mask it with drugs. Only dentists can change the skeleton of the head by permanently changing the orthopedic structural support pillars and guidance systems of the skeleton of the jaws and head: the teeth, lack of teeth, and poor alignment. By altering the skeleton via the teeth, dentists are able to stop and prevent the neuromuscular and orthopedic assaults on both the TNS and the TMJoints from returning. It's a permanent change to the skeleton that improves the function of the joints and relieves stresses on the TNS.

Does it scare you to know doctors aren't making the decisions about what is best for the patient's health? Does it frighten you to know that administrators who don't have medical degrees are making health decisions for you? It terrifies and angers me.

We've all heard the phrase "follow the money," and unfortunately for the patient, that saying applies all too well in this situation. If you are never properly examined for this problem, you will never be diagnosed or referred. Instead, you will be put on what feels like a merry-go-round—going from doctor to doctor in the same clinic or network. Eventually, this merry-go-round becomes a whirlpool that sucks you into a cesspool of chronic, hellish pain where you incur excessive medical bills. All the while, too many sectors of the medical and pharmaceutical industries get rich.

I've experienced the exclusivity and irrationality of in-house operations firsthand. I've spoken three times at one of the largest medical clinics in the Milwaukee area about TMJ, TNS-related pain, and the treatments I offer for chronic pain. I explained our success rate for eliminating chronic pain symptoms without drugs. On one occasion, my opening slide even offered a money-back guarantee if we could not eliminate a patient's recurring migraines or tension headaches.

Five staff members from the clinic came in for treatment, and each

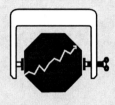

NEWSWORTHY TRUTH

If you are never properly examined for this problem, you will never be diagnosed or referred. Instead, you will be put on what feels like a merry-go-round—going from doctor to doctor in the same "in-house" clinic or network.

one improved by 80 to 100 percent. Amazingly, only one doctor ever referred any patients to me—and that particular doctor is a friend and patient of mine. Does that mean the rest of the doctors at this clinic don't encounter patients who suffer from debilitating migraines or other chronic pain symptoms? Unlikely. Headaches and neck pain are among the top reasons people go to see their physicians.

There have been many books and articles addressing the problems of greed and inadequate care resulting from in-house operations. Even with the level of scrutiny and transparency that the Internet and social media bring to the situation, physicians are still allowed to let patients suffer. They are permitted, even encouraged, not to examine patients for the underlying cause of their pain, or refer in network even if that particular doctor/dentist doesn't have a great track record for producing pain-free results.

WHAT IS AT STAKE FOR PHARMACEUTICAL COMPANIES?

"My husband and I really thought I was going to die. My pain was so intense that I didn't work for about a year. I just went from doctor to doctor. It was so frustrating. Insurance kept sending us from one specialist to another, and no one was able to diagnose what was going on.

We found Dr. Seymour on the Internet. It was splint therapy that ended up curing my symptoms. I started to feel better in two-and-a-half weeks. It's like night and day now. I'm back to normal and our family life is back to normal.

I was shocked to find out the insurance companies didn't have to cover this. I don't need the pain medications. I don't need all the medications the doctors prescribed and I don't even need sleep medication anymore. I have no more symptoms. I feel wonderful."

—A.S., former chronic pain sufferer

The pharmaceutical Goliaths have so much money it's difficult to estimate their power. In fact, I chose to self-publish this book because I felt certain that this mega-industry wields its control over a number of publishing companies. Dr. Marcia Angell's book, *The Truth About the Drug Companies: How They Deceive Us and What to Do About It*, explains how widespread Big Pharma's (nickname given to the pharmaceutical industry) influence extends. In 2002, for example, the top ten drug companies in the United States on the Fortune 500 Companies list earned more in profits than the other 490 companies together. To get the true scope of that statement, you must understand that list includes the oil companies, energy companies, and General Motors. The biggest companies in the world added all together and the drug companies' profits still exceed the other 490 companies. That adds up to a great deal of influence that, as Dr. Angell points out, is very difficult to trace.

I believe pharmaceutical companies, pharmacies and pharmacists all share part of the blame in the perpetuation of this prison of pain. In essence, prescription drugs can be a double-edged sword. On the good side, they provide some pain relief for those who might otherwise be unable to cope with day-to-day life. On the bad side, patients are robbed of long-term, drug-free solutions because far too much money is at stake. It only makes financial sense that pharmacies and the pharmaceutical industry don't want to give up enormous profits they earn off chronic pain patients. Many of the patients who come to see us at the Chronic Pain Solution Center are already on a drug regimen that costs more than $1,000 per month. In most cases, insurance companies cover approximately 80 percent, leaving patients with a $200 monthly bill for medication. Fees for multiple doctor visits and tests as well as monthly insurance premiums bite even deeper into the patient's wallet. If there are 30 million migraine patients in the United States alone, and if only half of them have a monthly drug bill of $1,000, that computes to $15 billion per month—$180 billion per year—going to pharmaceutical companies. Beyond the risk of losing money on pain medication, these companies also stand to see a decrease in sales of anti-anxiety, antidepressant, chronic fatigue, vertigo, muscle relaxant, and sleep medications.

Like doctors and insurance carriers, researchers and executives at pharmaceutical companies have known for decades that the trigeminal nerve system is a major contributor to migraine headaches. Remember,

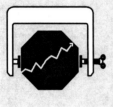

NEWSWORTHY TRUTH

Like doctors and insurance carriers, researchers and executives at pharmaceutical companies have known for decades that the trigeminal nerve system is a major contributor to migraine headaches.

studies through the centuries have connected headaches to the teeth. Certainly in the past fifty to one hundred years, professional articles and books have explained the connection between the TNS, TMJ, and the teeth with migraines and recurring headaches. These giants are also aware that TMJoint appliance therapy successfully relieves some of these headaches without drugs, yet these companies do very little with their billions of research and development funds to study and create better, longer-lasting devices and preventive studies regarding the TNS and TMJoints. The pharmaceutical giants give the National Headache Foundation over $1 million for research, yet the NHF does little to nothing to study appliance therapy. Its materials devote precious little space to the TNS and TMJoints as a cause of headaches. And why not? Week after week, patients visit their clinics for extensive, expensive testing. These patients leave with a list of foods and beverages to avoid and suggested lifestyle changes—and prescriptions for multiple drugs. What would an organization that promotes prescriptions so effectively be worth to drug companies? Remember: Drugs mask the problem; they don't treat the cause.

I believe without reservation that the TNS and TMJoints are the primary causes of migraines and all types of headaches. Our success rate for treatment and relief would not be as high as it is *without drugs* if these physical structures weren't the major cause.

Pharmacies and our pharmacists are part of the system that perpetuates the practice of pain for profit. Over the years, I've also treated pharmacists and the spouses of pharmacists. They have benefited from the drug- and surgery-free treatment offered at my clinic, and yet not one of them would be allowed to refer anyone else to me without endangering their jobs. Believe me, I've asked for referrals. But the responses always fall into one of two categories:

- I'd be fired for cutting off an income source of over a thousand dollars a month to the pharmacy.
- I would be referring the patient away from one of our network of physicians.

Again, just as in the medical clinics, patient treatment decisions are handed down by administrators or owners of the pharmacy, as dictated by their bottom line.

Believe it or not, I've actually had a pharmacy contact my clinic after we eliminated a patient's migraines, and request that we recommend the patient to continue her expensive preventive migraine medication. They didn't just send a letter; they included a bibliography, listing three articles *sponsored by drug companies.* Wow! That letter was addressed to the Chronic Pain *Solution* Center. I wonder what they think Solution means? In my book, solution doesn't mean a regimen of costly and potentially harmful drugs.

I know many chronic pain suffers could not have continued living without the temporary relief some prescriptions offer. When you are in agony, you will take whatever doctors prescribe to make the pain stop. But if you're kept on drugs long term without anyone telling you about treatments that can potentially *eliminate* your pain and the need to take these medicines, are they really helping you as they should? Bottom-line medicine is in line with your best interests. If information has been out there about the successful treatment of migraines and headaches relative to TMJoints and the TNS for years, decades, or centuries, don't you think someone should be telling you about it? Instead, there is an entire industry earning hundreds of billions of dollars per year off your pain and suffering. According to Dr. Marcia Angell's book, these massive pharmaceutical companies are so powerful they can control which articles are published in medical journals. They put people on medical school boards and influence what students are taught. They also wield significant power within the FDA (Food and Drug Administration) and Congress. The pharmaceutical industry actually has more lobbyists on Capitol Hill than there are legislators. I'm a firm believer in capitalism, but I also know it breaks down when companies are permitted to have unlimited lobbyists to promote their financial interests, rather than the interests of those they are supposed to be helping.

Some skeptics may try to shift attention and claim that I am promoting this treatment and demanding that insurance companies cover it for my own financial gain. The truth is, I and other trained dentists will benefit financially when doctors are forced to examine, diagnose and refer patients for TMJ- and TNS-related pain, especially if insurance companies are rightfully required to cover their clients for the necessary treatment. The difference between the pharmaceutical companies and us at the Chronic Pain Solution Center is that the pharmaceutical companies get paid to keep covering up the painful symptoms. We, on the other hand, *eliminate the cause of your pain so you no longer need pain medications or migraine prevention drugs for life.*

Does it Make Sense to Mask Pain?

Imagine that every day on your way into work you had a choice between two doors. One door is so short you hit your head on the top every time you went through it. The other offers plenty of clearance. Would you continue to go through the door where you kept hitting your head and simply take medication to cover up the pain of your growing head trauma and abuse? Or would you find a way to avoid the cause by going through another door or making the door taller? The drug companies choose to *cover up the pain and let the damage continue.* Of course, it takes physicians to write the prescriptions for all these pain meds. It is in the pharmaceutical company's interest to entice physicians as well as large medical and pain clinics with perks and benefits to ensure their prescriptions are written.

But doctors aren't the only ones pharmaceutical companies woo. Look at TV. At one time, cigarette ads were pervasive. "Once upon a time, drug companies promoted drugs to treat diseases. Now it is often the opposite. They promote diseases to fit their drugs," writes Angell in *The Truth about Drug Companies,* "Nearly everyone experiences heartburn from time to time. The remedy used to be a glass of milk or an over-the-counter antacid to relieve the symptoms. But now heartburn is called 'acid reflux disease' or 'gastroesophageal reflux disease (GERD)' and marketed, along with the drugs to treat it, as a harbinger of serious esophageal disease—which it usually is not. As a result, in 2002, Prilosec was the third best-selling drug in the world (Nexium had not yet had a chance to replace it), and its competitor Prevacid was seventh."

Boniva is another drug to watch out for. They have sweet Sally Fields, *The Flying Nun* (TV series from 1967–1970), sell you on preventing osteoporosis, not mentioning that it causes necrosis of the jaw and premature hip fractures. Unfortunately, the focus has shifted from finding a cure to finding markets and selling drugs. Pharmaceutical companies have become masters at pitching drugs that offer questionable benefits and significant, detrimental side effects... even when natural and safe treatments are available.

Drug companies are not the Good Samaritans they would have you believe in their rampant commercials. Before you go on any drug long term, research the disease, preventive methods, and the side effects of the prescribed drug. As with the milk antidote for heartburn, natural or non-drug solutions often exists. And certainly, by now you realize a long-term, drug-free solution is available for most types of headaches. Now, if we can just get the word out past the pharmaceutical companies.

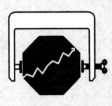

NEWSWORTHY TRUTH

Pharmaceutical companies have become masters at pitching drugs that offer questionable benefits and significant, detrimental side effects... even when natural and safe treatments are available.

You know the old joke: What does the eight hundred pound gorilla do? *Anything it wants to.* What's true of the eight hundred pound gorilla is true of the Colossus that is the pharmaceutical industry. It is used to doing pretty much what it wants to do. It will continue to do so until the public—millions of people like you and me—stand up and demand better. If this is ever going to change we must all confront our doctors (including all specialists) who prescribe long-term drug solutions. It must become unacceptable that the only option for better health and well being comes from a pill. Be willing to take the necessary step of seeking out a doctor who can treat the source of your pain rather than simply mask it with drugs.

One of the most important things you can do is share what you've learned in this book with *everyone* you know. Pharmaceutical companies have billions of dollars at their disposal to persuade public opinion. We have something better: millions/billions of people who should be very angry at the truth that these companies and doctors have been intentionally keeping them dependent on strong pain medications, muscle relaxants, antidepressants, anxiety and sleep medications. It can't be said often enough that women must use the Internet as a means to distribute information worldwide and create a flood of insight. We must demand that instead of researching ways to keep you coming back, that the research shifts to creating even better orthotics and even more precise technology to help eliminate and prevent chronic pain and migraines. When is the last time you saw a fundraiser to end migraines and chronic tension headaches that involved a study related to the teeth and TMJoints, or TNS? It's important to remember that the connection has been known and written about since the 1700s and 1800s.

Make no mistake: These companies will not back off without a fight. Keeping you and millions like you in pain is how they stay in business.

Why Do Insurance Companies Deny Coverage?

In December 2010, my health began to deteriorate. I experienced bouts of severe vertigo accompanied by tingling sensations in the back of my head as well as down both of my arms and into my hands and fingers. The vertigo was so bad I had to crawl on my belly just to get to the restroom. I went to an urgent care clinic two or three times before Christmas. After several series of tests, CT scans, x-rays, and antibiotics, I was told I was just stressed out and was prescribed more medication for anti-anxiety and depression.

Frustrated and feeling desperate and miserable, I typed my symptoms into Google. I was stunned to see that everything I was experiencing was described on websites for TMJ disorder. We called all of the in-network oral surgeons but they said they no longer treat TMJ patients.

Finally, a friend told me about Dr. Seymour. After tests and x-rays, he found that my right jaw was dislocated, and I suffered terribly from TMJ disorder. I began splint therapy. It took several weeks and a lot of pain as my jaw began to move, but now, nine months later, I can honestly say that I am 100 percent better, and no longer have any of the symptoms I had before going to see Dr. Seymour.

My temporary splint is made of plastic so it wears down quickly, and each time I need to go in for repair, it is costly. That is why Dr. Seymour is ready for me to move on to what he calls Phase Two treatment to re-adjust my bite so the symptoms do not return. My insurance company will not help pay for my treatment because Dr. Seymour is out of network. We called the in-network specialists and found only one that treats TMJ. He is a surgeon who would have to start treating me as a new patient, more than likely using surgery as treatment.

Why should I have to start over and risk having my health regress when I have found a doctor who can treat me without surgery? Why would an insurance company be willing to pay more for surgery than for crowns or prosthesis?

We have piles of doctor bills that have accumulated since last December, including a huge bill from early spring when the stress of this situation caused me to be hospitalized due to pain, stress, depression, and anxiety. I cannot continue with Phase Two because we simply cannot afford to pay for it out of pocket ourselves. With all of this waiting, the bills are continuing to mount and are causing me more stress. The expense of medications to handle that is adding up.

—D.K ., Pain for profit victim

TWENTY-FIVE YEARS AGO, ONE OF MY PATIENTS, AN ENGINEER, WAS TOLD HE NEEDED BACK SURGERY. One of his legs was shorter than the other and discrepancy caused a great deal of back pain. His doctor was ready to operate and his insurance company was lined up to pay for the surgery, but he thought, "If I were dealing with a beam in a building, I'd simply increase the height of the shorter beam by putting a shim (wedge) under it." He had a shoemaker design a wedge to his specifications to go under the heel of his shoe and make both legs equal lengths. Using common sense and basic engineering, my patient did something very similar to what we do in the mouth. From his engineering background he recognized that what I was doing to increase the height of some of the teeth in his wife's mouth was similar to what he did to make his leg lengths equal. By balancing the skeleton of the head (the teeth), we can prevent the weight shift that forward head posture causes and avoid painful and costly surgeries. Today, twenty-five years later, both he and his wife are happy and healthy because we balanced the skeleton of his wife's head and upper body via the teeth, just as he balanced his lower skeleton upward via leg length. She's been pain-free and drug-free for decades, and he's never had to have back surgery.

It seems simple and straightforward, right? It's a matter of common sense. So why is it that, time and again, after insurance companies have progress reports signed by the patient proving they are 80 percent pain-free without drugs while on the Phase One diagnostic orthotic, these major medical insurance companies are permitted to deny these women their medical rights to have the long-term cure? How can it possibly be true that thousands of dollars a year in major medical insurance premiums do not provide coverage for such a vital joint and a nerve that surrounds the brain? Now, recognize again the fact that the orthotic has proven for this patient that the treatment works. Why would they not want to permanently alter the skeleton, improve the head posture, and relieve pain *without* the expense of surgery, eliminating decades of $1,000 per month payments in pharmaceutical bills and psychiatric help?

The only answer I've been able to come up with is money. Here is the problem: The money giants of the medical and pharmaceutical industries dictate medical insurance coverage. The same people who rake in a half-trillion dollars per year off the chronic suffering of women and the elderly determine what gets covered. They will do everything possible to dictate that dental treatments for chronic pain and migraines are not covered, even though dentistry is the only profession truly trained to alter the teeth permanently and treat this problem. It's like putting the fox in charge of the chicken coop.

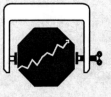

NEWSWORTHY TRUTH

Millions of patients—three out of every four of whom are women—are condemned to a life of suffering unless they can afford to pay for the treatment out of pocket.

Other treatments, including the surgeries, endless drugs, and chiropractic appointments are covered by insurance. Medicare will only cover the problem if the dentist is a Medicare provider. Unfortunately, the amount Medicare covers for the disorder doesn't compensate auxiliary staff salaries, let alone expenses related to extra space and specialized diagnostic computer and x-ray equipment.

In essence, millions of patients—three out of every four of whom are women—are condemned to a life of suffering unless they can afford to pay for the treatment out of pocket. This pain-for-profit epidemic is exacerbated by the "in-house" policies that drive our medical and insurance system.

A SHORT-LIVED VICTORY

In 1997, the Wisconsin Dental Association (WDA) and I went to the state capital to get the legislature to mandate major medical insurance companies to cover treatment for TMJ-related pain. (You'll read more about this in Chapter Eleven, "What Are Dentists Doing to Help the Issue?") We were successful in getting that bill passed, limited as it may be, but only because the governor had promised his dentist he would sign the bill if we were able to get it through the committees and onto his desk. (Five years earlier, the governor had vetoed a similar bill.) Leaders of the WDA and I were elated with the strides we had made on behalf of countless suffering patients, but our victory was short-lived. Two months after coverage of TMJ disorders was mandated, the legislature—feeling the pressure of the HMO insurance companies' lobbyists—capped the annual coverage for treating one of the most complex joints in the entire body at $1,250.

If you can possibly imagine this, after we were able to prove to patients and their insurance companies using the temporary Phase One orthotic that this treatment will relieve their pain without drugs or surgery, the insurance companies still do not have to cover any portion of the cost of the permanent solution. The permanent treatment, Phase Two, consists of permanently restoring the proper height, guidance and engineering of the skeletal support pillars of the bite (the teeth) using partial dentures and fixed bridges to replace missing teeth, crowns to increase the height of teeth, correct poor alignment and guidance systems, or simply bonding, on guidance and balancing bite on the Tekscan bite computer. It's like saying to a cancer patient or heart patient: *We know of a treatment that will solve your problem, but we don't have anyone "in house" who can do this. It's too expensive (and it doesn't require a $1,000 monthly bill) and it's dental. It's not really medical so you're going to have to go back to suffering.* Can you think of anything more ridiculous? Nothing was permanently changed in Phase One; the lack of support that caused the problem in the first place still exists. The temporary plastic orthotic cannot endure forces of the magnitude in the posterior of the mouth (hundreds of pounds per square inch) for more than six months to a year and continue to provide the needed vertical support.

The denial of coverage for the long-term solution that has proven to the patient and the insurance company that it eliminates their pain without drugs, illustrates just how little insurance companies care about helping the people find relief from chronic suffering. It has been four-teen years since the passage of this bill in the state of Wisconsin, and although we've repeatedly proven the effectiveness of this treatment to a number of insurance companies, they still refuse to cover the long-term solution to the pain. They, in fact, do not appear to be at all interested in the results we are able to achieve, or in the treatments we use to relieve so many patients of tension headaches, migraines, and other chronic pain symptoms.

'A LOW-TICKET ITEM'

A few years ago, an insurance company attempted to reclaim $70,000 they had paid me for treating patients approximately three to four years earlier. If you can believe it, one of the patients for whom they decided to reclaim payments was the woman who had migraines for sixty-four years before coming to our clinic. Their customers (my patients) were living pain-free and were very satisfied with the results of the treatment I had provided them. But the insurance company reviewed its files and decided dentists shouldn't be treating patients for migraines. To set the scales back in its favor, the insurance company began withholding funds due on claims of current patients.

I contacted the insurance company's attorney to discuss the issue. In a moment of clarity and utter honesty, the attorney said, "It appears that you have an excellent treatment for migraine headaches, and it is low-ticket item compared to the other treatments out there." (Not surprisingly, I have not been able to reach that attorney at the company since then. I hope he didn't lose his job.) His acknowledgment is as close as I have come to hearing from any insurance employee that they noticed how effective this treatment is based on our patients' progress reports.

An attorney friend from my church advised me against hiring an attorney and taking the company to court, "Their corporate attorneys will bleed you dry," he predicted. So instead, I prayed about the matter and wrote the company a long letter citing ten cases of patients they covered who had suffered for years with migraines. I included progress reports showing how each of these patients had improved dramatically under my care. I also quoted their attorney who had remarked that this treatment is both effective and comparatively inexpensive. With God, the One who called me to get involved in all this back in 1974, as my attorney, I also cited James 3:5 from the Message translation of the Bible:

"A word out of your mouth may seem of no account, but it can accomplish nearly anything—or destroy it! It only takes a spark, remember, to set off a forest fire." I signed off with this statement, "I have been looking for the spark to start this forest fire for thirty years. If this be the spark, bring it."

God, my Attorney, came through. A month later I received a letter from the company stating that it was not going to pursue the $70,000. The insurance company backed off (which is why I chose not to name it in this book); however, I never received the first few thousand it withheld from my other patients' claims.

If this were a poker game, I would call the company's decision to back off a "tell," a poker term for a tip-off of weakness. I believe that company—and the industry as whole—is afraid of the repercussions of this information getting out. These companies fully understand the potential for this "low-ticket" item and for some reasons (I would love to know who's controlling the insurance companies) they are content with a system that keeps patients in pain for decades. At the same time, I realize that I am risking everything by working to get this message and the amazing truth about Headfirst Preventative Medicine out to the public. But I ask you, what would you do if you were sixty-six years old, and roadblock after roadblock had been set up against what was successful for thirty-eight years at eliminating 80 percent of the pain in 80 to 95 percent of the cases you see? What action would you take if you were certain you had information and proof of a treatment that could help billions of pain prisoners around the world, but people kept telling you, "there's no way you can ever get this done in your lifetime"? Relieving people from chronic pain is my calling. And this insurance company's "tell" confirms that I'm on the right track. I hope that you'll join me in this mission to change the way the insurance and medical industries not only treat this problem, but, more importantly, how they treat you!

THE MEDICAL INSURANCE LOOPHOLE

The chronic pain and migraines discussed in this book are an orthopedic (joint, muscles, and bones) and neurologic (TNS) problem. But because the teeth are the only place the skeleton comes through the skin allowing us to permanently decompress the joints (separate the two bones by making the teeth taller) and then prevent the bones from rubbing on the nerves (TNS) to get rid of the pain, the insurance companies label it a dental problem. They are allowed to deny medical coverage for any symptom they can tie back to the TNS by identifying the issue as a TMJ problem. And TMJoints are not covered across the board. How ridiculous it this?

Here's how it works, or rather, doesn't work when a patient comes into the clinic suffering with stabbing eye pain that feels like a "hot poker or ice pick in the eye." We know that one of the three major branches of the TNS, the ophthalmic branch, is a sensory nerve that supplies the eyes. (Note that the name for eye specialists, ophthalmologists, derives from the same name give to the upper branch of the TNS.) If we treat and eliminate that pain using an orthotic that covers the teeth to eliminate numerous traumatic assaults on the TNS, the insurance company doesn't care that the pain is gone. They deny coverage simply because a "TMJ treatment" was used.

The same holds true for the patient who has stabbing ear pain. If she goes to an ENT (ear, nose and throat specialist) who performs surgery to treat the TNS, that surgery is covered. In many cases, her pain can be relieved using a non-surgical orthotic treatment that insurance companies will not cover. The scenario is repeated time and again. Surgeries performed on the neck, sinuses, and the trigeminal nerve itself to attempt to relieve neck pain, migraines, tension headaches, sinus pain, and trigeminal neuralgia are all covered by insurance, and they are far more expensive than this treatment. What's worse, they don't correct the problem because they're not treating the cause and the pain returns. The

TNS is involved in every case, which means a non-surgical treatment is very likely available. At a minimum, the non-surgical approach should be explored first. But the non-surgical treatment is classified as a TMJ issue, and medical insurance denies the claim.

You see, most health insurance policies include a clause that says the TMJoints are not covered. You read that right. These companies are permitted not to cover joints that are vital to your survival. I'm sure when you took out your health insurance, you assumed if it covered your knee, hip, ankle, and shoulder joints, it would also cover your jaw joints as part of the body that you are paying exorbitant monthly premiums to cover. But in more than half of the states in the union, TMJoints are not covered by major medical insurance. As a result, people end up living with horrendous pain. It's like buying a car and asking "Does it come with the engine, or do I have to buy that separately?" A car won't run without an engine, and you can't survive well without functioning TMJoints. Yes, you could have intravenous feedings, or go on a soft-food diet forever, but is that living? And is that what you thought you were paying premiums for?

STUNTS INSURANCE COMPANIES PULL

In defense of dentistry, the stunts that insurance companies pull are a major reason that there aren't more dentists diagnosing and treating chronic pain. We do our part as professionals by documenting our patients' progress. To speed the payment process, our practice sends copies of progress reports filled out and signed by the patients themselves to show how the treatment has worked or is working. Even with this documentation, insurance providers typically respond to their clients' (our patients') claims using creative tactics like these:

- They tell the patient they are applying the treatment toward their deductible, but never ask for notes relative to the type of treatment. Once the deductible is met they ask for all notes to be copied and sent. Then they deny the claim. *If the treatment was not going to be covered, the patient and our office should have been informed on the first visit.*

- One insurance company paid all of a patient's claims for a year of treatment only to turn around the following year and request that the money be repaid!

- Customer service calls get diverted to outsourced call centers. In one case, we were given four different rapid-resolution numbers. The company indicated it would settle the claims in seven to ten business days. The rapid resolution number was a complete scam; eighteen months later, not one of the claims was settled.

A Typical Waste of Time

One of the first questions my team asks when we appeal these cases for our clients with the insurance company board is: "What is your medical experience?"

In almost every case, no one on the board has any medical experience.

Now understand that as the patient's care-giver, I have taken time out of my schedule to be on this call. Members of my staff have also taken time out of their workday. That means my office is losing both time and money to participate in this call.

The board typically offers to set up another conference so a physician can be on the call—inconveniencing and costing everyone productive time out of their day once again. The physician they hire for the call generally knows very little about this treatment to begin with, and is undoubtedly trained or coerced into saying the word DENIED. Which is exactly what they do even after we endure all their antics.

- Language barriers at offsite call centers prevent communication and progress. Eventually, the agent supplies yet another "rapid resolution" number.

- Sometimes the insurance company refers claims to a third party for resolution… and they own the third party.

- Often we will send multiple pages of records to the insurance company for multiple dates. We will get calls with requests for records or x-rays that we've already sent. They received some, but claim to be missing other documents, even though all the documents were sent in the same envelope.

- Or my favorite example of avoiding their client's needs is when the agent gives us the wrong number to reach a supervisor. If that happened only once or twice I'd chalk it up to a mistake. But this is a repetitive practice.

The ploys used by the insurance companies never cease to amaze me or the patient, and they keep coming up with new ones. I've even had insurance company "deniers" go after my professional license. Blue Cross Blue Shield and Humana have tried to go after my license saying I was not authorized to use codes that I was treating migraines via the TNS. They lost in all cases. This proves that the licensing board agrees that I have the right to treat migraines and all these symptoms that are related to the trigeminal nerve with my dental license! Now explain this: I've met with the Commissioner of Insurance for the state of Wisconsin, I've won the licensing issue, they all agree I have the right to treat this; but no one has the power to make the insurance companies cover this treatment. How ridiculous! It is going to be up to the women and elderly from this point as to how long they're allowed to get away with allowing you to suffer for decades.

This is the important part of this story for those of you who still think insurance companies care about you. In every case, these "deniers" have progress reports filled out and signed by the patients stating they were at least 80 percent better without drugs. Why would insurance companies take the doctor who was healing patients to the licensing board, and *not touch the thousands of doctors who are doing nothing to diagnose or treat the problem?* The only reason I can come up with is money. When patients are kept suffering, the "money train" keeps chugging along — fueled by a half-trillion dollars per year in surgeries and treatments that don't work or keep you coming back for temporary relief and drugs that mask the problem year after year.

UPFRONT COSTS VS. LONG-TERM SAVINGS

From a business standpoint, what sense does it make for insurance companies to exclude TMJoints from coverage and consistently deny claims that offer long-term relief? Sure, restoring teeth and re-engineering mouths come with upfront costs, but this non-invasive treatment eliminates countless surgeries, drug expenses and side effects, and decades of doctor visits. Take a look at the findings and implications of this disorder as laid out by studies conducted by the Blue Cross Blue Shield HMO, TMJ experts, and the World Health Organization. Let's start with a study conducted by a major player in the insurance industry.

In a 1998 article in *The Journal of Craniomandibular Practice* titled "Health Care Utilization by Patients With Temporomandibular Joint Disorders,"[18] Dr. Daniel D. Shimshak and Maureen C. Defer reported on a major study done by an HMO of Blue Cross Blue Shield. It compared the overall cost of health care for thousands of TMJ patients versus non-TMJ patients in regard to outpatient, inpatient, psychiatric, as well as age and sex variables. Their findings were astounding.

Their study found that patients with TMJ disorders went to doctors and healthcare facilities much more than non-TMJ patients. Not surprisingly, claims directly associated with complaints about the TMJoint itself were very small because patients rarely experience pain in the joint itself. Symptoms of this disorder generally show up as referred pain, including headaches, neck and back pain, chronic depression, anxiety, sleep disorders, and chronic fatigue, etc. This truth is why the cost of covering a patient with TMJ problems was much higher than non-TMJ subjects. For some of the major diagnostic categories, such as nervousness (headaches qualify here), respiratory, circulatory, and digestive issues, the inpatient and outpatient claim differences in healthcare visits, testing, and all variables included were as high as three times the costs for non-TMJ patients across the board. And with the effects that this problem has on sense of balance, light sensitivity, and night driving, I'm not at all surprised these patients are more apt to suffer accidents and trauma at a much higher rate than non-TMJ patients.

The HMO study found only one category, pregnancy and childbirth, where costs were greater for non-TMJ than for subjects who were TMJ patients. Healthcare costs for pregnancy and childbirth for patients *without* a TMJ or chronic pain problem are 2.5 times that of TMJ sufferers. (See the table on p. 174.) This ties directly into the age-old statement, "Honey I have a headache." Women who are in pain most of the time due to this problem are much less likely to feel well enough to consider having sex, let alone having more children to care for.

Additionally, the costs for psychiatric care were found to be at least twice that of those of non-TMJ subjects. Claims related to psychiatric benefits fall into two categories, mental and alcohol and drug abuse. The lack of coverage contributes to the alcohol and drug abuse over all. Without viable treatment, many chronic pain patients go to extreme measures to find relief. I believe psychiatric care is much higher than the HMO study revealed. So many patients who come into our clinic have lost the support of their husbands, family and friends to the point that they are thought of as hypochondriacs. Also, many psychiatric appointments would not have been reported in this study because patients had to go outside the HMO network coverage and pay for them out of pocket.

Cost Differences for Patients with TMJ Disorders

Inpatient Claims Distributed by MDC
Adjusted for Age and Sex

MDC	Admissions per 1000			Cost per capita		
	TMJ	Non-TMJ	% Difference	TMJ	Non-TMJ	% Difference
0 Missing/Invalid Diagnosis	0.00	0.01	-100.0	$ 0.00	$ 0.01	-100.0
1 Nervous	8.17	2.43	236.2	107.30	28.75	273.2
2 Eye	0.58	0.19	205.3	41.84	0.95	4304.2
3 Ear/Nose/Mouth/Throat	16.93	1.14	1385.1	159.34	4.71	3283.0
4 Respiratory	6.42	4.21	52.5	65.37	29.08	124.8
5 Circulatory	12.26	7.20	70.3	89.09	64.50	38.1
6 Digestive	8.76	6.01	45.8	58.17	40.80	42.6
7 Liver/Pancreas	4.67	2.84	64.4	26.16	21.91	19.4
8 Musculoskeletal	6.42	5.13	25.1	58.53	43.98	33.1
9 Skin Breast	4.67	2.14	118.2	31.03	14.61	112.4
10 Metabolic	1.17	1.54	-24.0	3.07	10.22	-70.0
11 Kidney	2.92	1.96	49.0	41.84	12.00	248.7
12 Male Reproductive	0.58	0.35	65.7	2.60	2.85	-8.8
13 Female Reproductive	5.25	4.13	27.1	25.38	26.09	-2.7
14 Pregnancy/Childbirth	13.43	32.16	-58.2	62.48	156.69	-60.1
15 Newborns	0.00	3.51	-100.0	0.00	11.18	-100.0
16 Blood	0.00	0.42	-100.0	0.00	5.12	-100.0
17 Spine/Bone Marrow	4.09	1.27	222.0	20.87	15.52	34.5
18 Infections	2.92	0.94	210.6	14.19	7.08	100.4
19 Mental*	1.17	1.00	17.0	3.38	5.15	-34.4
20 Alcohol/Drug Use*	1.17	0.56	108.9	9.87	1.32	647.7
21 Injuries/Poisonings	1.75	0.94	86.2	7.72	3.92	96.9
22 Burns	0.00	0.04	-100.0	0.00	0.52	-100.0
23 Health Status	0.58	0.27	114.8	1.27	4.00	-68.3
24 Multiple Trauma	1.75	0.14	1150.0	86.37	3.37	2462.9
25 HIV Infections	1.75	0.17	929.4	19.98	2.41	729.0
Totals	107.41	80.70	33.1	$935.86	$516.74	81.1

*Excludes claims processed by designated psychiatric benefits vendor

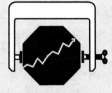

NEWSWORTHY TRUTH

An HMO study revealed how much more people with TMJ disorder cost insurance companies.

- Inpatient claims and admissions costs were 81 percent higher.

- Outpatient costs for TMJ patients were 100 percent higher.

- Psychiatric care costs were double for TMJ patients.

The most dramatic differences in cost were associated with nervous disorders (headaches qualify here); eye, ear, nose, mouth and throat (all supplied by the TNS); circulatory; and multiple trauma categories.

(See the table on p. 174.)

In the April 2005 edition of *The Journal of Cranial Mandibular Practice* (a journal for dentists specializing in the treatment of chronic pain related to the TMJoints and TNS)[23], Dr. H. Clifton Simmons III states that Phase One orthotic therapy resulted in either total absence of pain or improvement by 95 percent of the symptoms present before treatment. Simmons notes, "TMJ disease should be highly placed in the differential diagnosis of patients presenting with these symptoms." In other words, TMJ disorders should be the first place we look when patients exhibit symptoms such as headache, neck pain, vertigo, sleep loss, chronic fatigue, and chronic depression. I'd go a step further and say that in no scenario should doctors be permitted to ignore these symptoms as potential side effects of TMJ and TNS pain. In addition to being required to examine for and diagnose TMJ and TNS issues, doctors and dentists must be required to refer patients to a trained dentist who can actually treat the issue. Keeping patients "In-House" only prolongs the pain.

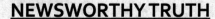

NEWSWORTHY TRUTH

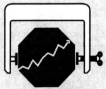

The World Health Organization (WHO)[24] reiterates the prevalence of this epidemic and the need for a cure. A fact sheet published by WHO outlines ways headaches cause impaired quality of life and financial burdens. Although this document specifically addresses headaches, by now you understand that the list of symptoms tied into the TNS is much more extensive. WHO lists such issues as:

- Substantial personal suffering,

- Repeated headache attacks combined with the constant fear of the next one,

- Damaged family life, social life and employment,

- Predisposition of individuals dealing long-term with chronic headaches to other illnesses and substantial levels of disability,

- Greater healthcare costs in general,

- Three times the risk for chronic depression,

- Reduced social activity and work capacity.

WHO also recognizes facts previously mentioned in this book:

- Headaches and migraines commonly start at puberty.

- Three times more European and American women than men suffer from migraines.

- Headache disorders are disabling. WHO lists headaches as one of the top ten most disabling conditions for the two genders, and *one of the top five most disabling for women*.

- A minority of people with headache disorders worldwide are diagnosed appropriately by a healthcare provider.

A fact sheet on headaches published by the World Health Organization (WHO) states: **"Headache disorders are among the most common disorders of the nervous system. They are pandemic and, in many cases, life-long conditions."** This international health organization recognizes that headaches are a burden of *pandemic* proportions. This burden, it notes, is "sufficient to justify a strategic change in the approach to headache management." It's time our insurance companies acknowledge this truth as well!

Headaches are one of the most common symptoms for which people go to the doctor, yet physicians have very little training regarding headaches and their causes. "A survey of neurologists found that up to one-third of all their patients consulted them because of headache—more than for any other complaint," WHO states. Still, the cause remains unrecognized and undertreated worldwide.

The document notes that headache or facial pain can be attributed to disorders of the cranium, neck, eyes, ears, nose, sinuses, teeth, mouth or other facial or cranial structures (the exact list of structures that the TNS supplies). And although headaches rarely signal serious underlying illness, physicians consistently order MRIs and expensive tests without performing a simple exam of structures irritating the TNS.

It also recognizes the high prevalence of headaches in Third World countries, as well as the economic costs in the United Kingdom. Twenty-five million work or school days are lost every year in the United Kingdom because of migraines alone. It's interesting to note that extractions are common in the UK.

"A survey of neurologists found that up to one-third of all their patients consulted them because of headache—
more than for any other complaint."
—World Health Organization

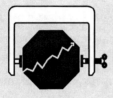

NEWSWORTHY TRUTH

If specially trained dentists were empowered to treat chronic pain via the TNS and TMJoint and eliminated the need for $1,000 per month in drugs for only one thousand people (a very conservative number), insurance companies could save **$1 million on patient drug costs per month, potentially for *decades*.**

The document goes on to say, "Headache ought to be a public health concern. Yet there is good evidence that very large numbers of people troubled by headache do not receive effective care…. Its public-health importance lies in its causal association with these personal and societal burdens of pain, disability, damaged quality of life and financial cost."

Those financial costs include not only the significant burden to the affected individual and her family (remember, three times as many women as men suffer from these debilitating symptoms), but also society as a whole. "Because headache disorders are most troublesome in the productive years, late teens to 50s, estimates of their financial cost to society principally from lost working hours and reduced productivity are massive," notes WHO.

A cure is available for this largely female pandemic of pain. My hope is that organizations like WHO will get behind this message and promote this cure. The effort begins by spreading the word and forcing health professionals worldwide to diagnose and refer for treatment, rather than go with the status quo of ignoring the cause and masking the symptoms with drug after drug.

Let's circle back to the question at hand: Why would insurance companies fight covering the cost of treatment for TMJ disorders that would finally put an end to the pain, the drugs, the repeated office visits and adjustments, the testing, the surgeries and going from doctor to doctor? You would think they'd welcome any treatment that would end their payouts for all of these covered expenses, but instead they fight it like the plague.

POTENTIAL COST *SAVINGS* FOR INSURANCE COMPANIES

If specially trained dentists around the country were empowered to treat chronic pain via the TNS and TMJoint and eliminated the need for $1,000 per month in drugs for only one thousand people (a very conservative number), insurance companies could save $1 million on patient drug costs per month, potentially for decades.

Currently, 36 million people suffer from migraines in the United States. That number does not include the millions who suffer from chronic tension, cluster, and sinus headaches. Imagine the cost savings to insurance companies if dentists were empowered to treat these patients and relieve them of the need for migraine prescriptions. As stated earlier, many patients' medications cost upwards of $1,000 per month. Certainly not everyone is on that level of medication, so let's halve that number. If even 14.5 million people could get off their daily or monthly prescriptions, insurance companies could save $14.5 billion per month. The annual savings would be **$174 billion**. Multiply that number by the decades that many patients stay on migraine medications and the number is astronomical.

Pharmaceutical and insurance companies rely on these drug sales as guaranteed income. Case in point: CVS Pharmacy Insurance actually sent our clinic a letter recommending that a patient we had cured be put back on her preventive migraine meds, despite the fact that she no longer suffered from migraines and had no desire to take unnecessary medication. They sent that letter to our Chronic Pain *Solution* Center *without ever asking whether we provided a* **solution** *to end her headaches.*

Now consider this. The potential savings of $174 billion only takes into account Americans (not the billions worldwide who could similarly benefit from this treatment). Neither does his exorbitant number factor in the potential savings for insurance companies on treatments and doctor visits including:

- Regular doctor visits required to renew prescriptions,

- MRIs,

- CATscans,

- Other expensive neurologic testing that desperate patients undergo to find a cause and cure,

- Chiropractic or osteopathic adjustments (one to three times weekly),

- Acupuncturist appointments,

- Psychiatrist or psychologist appointments,

- Institutionalization of chronically depressed pain patients due to the long-term effects of chronic pain, chronic fatigue, malaise and side effects of drugs,

- Electric shock therapy in institutions,

- Ophthalmologist tests for the eye pain,

- ENT (ear, nose, throat) specialist appointments for chronic ear pain, hearing loss, vertigo (dizziness) and sinus problems,

- Expensive surgeries on the TN: Currently insurance covers $60,000 gamma knife surgeries for trigeminal neuralgia, to be followed up by more testing, but doesn't cover a simpler, far less expensive TMJ treatment.

- Emergency Room visits for even stronger drugs and overnight stays in the hospital,

- Week-long stays in the hospital and tests conducted by a panel of "specialists,"

- Extended stays in medical pain clinics or headache clinics at a cost of $20,000–30,000 per week,

- Costly and needless neck (cervical) fusions, conducted without ever putting a stethoscope on the TMJoint or measuring the opening and lateral movement of the lower jaw to determine if that is what's causing their forward and lateral head posture that is causing the neck pain,

- Shoulder surgeries,

- Sinus surgeries,

- Ear surgeries,

- Steroid injections into the openings between cervical vertebrae by anesthesiologists,

- Lower back operations due to forward and lateral head posture (curved spine) plus gravity, again conducted without examining for trauma to the TNS causing forward head posture,

- Surgeries on hips and knees and other weight-bearing joints caused by the forward head posture (curved spine),

- Sleep clinic testing and treatments for sleep apnea and sleep loss,

- Ulcerated stomachs and systemic operations that occur later in life due to all the strong and unnecessary medications patients ingest for years on end.

Does the practice of not covering relatively simple and inexpensive treatments make sense to you? When you look at the list above, can you see why I'm concerned about the primary motives of these insurance companies? Do you see why I say, "Follow the money"?

Across the board, the savings that insurance companies could realize by allowing trained dentists to treat and eliminate TNS- and TMJ-related pain is well into the hundreds of billions of dollars annually.[34] And yet, despite the savings they see from my patients who no longer need migraine medications and frequent doctor visits, they continue to deny claims.

The current system is not set up to benefit the patients. No, the winners here are the drug companies, the "in-house" clinics, hospitals and insurance companies that keep patients reliant on prescription

Pop Quiz

Here is a multiple choice quiz. Which of the following structures are not covered by major medical insurance?

A. The chief sensory nerve of the head and face,

B. The cranial nerve that has an effect on all five senses as well as the sense of balance,

C. Treatment that will stop muscle spasms in the strongest muscle of the body,

D. Treatment that will stop muscle spasms in the temporalis muscle that fans out over the entire temple area where many tension headaches and migraines originate,

E. Nonsurgical treatments for dislocated or arthritic jaw joints that are essential for life and are located just two millimeters from the floor of the brain.

Believe it or not, the answer is *all of the above*. All these important structures in the head and face are supposed to magically take care of themselves and are not covered by major medical insurance in twenty-eight out of fifty states, and poorly covered in the remaining twenty-two states.

medicines and so desperate for relief that they'll undergo any number of surgeries in hopes of finding a cure. Someone needs to figure out why insurance companies do not see the need to cover patients treated for TMJ and TNS disorders... and why they don't want to save billions of dollars per year by simply recognizing the field of Headfirst Preventative Medicine. I would imagine insurance company boardrooms are made up of physicians and representatives of the drug companies and rarely any dentists. The insurance debacle sounds bleak, but I believe that risk management departments of insurance companies will eventually require doctors to examine patients for problems related to the TNS and TMJ or risk being held liable for negligence... especially as they become aware of our mission to inform millions/billions of chronic pain sufferers of available treatment options.

Headfirst Preventive Medicine

If the skeleton of the head were examined first, rather than last or not at all, we could prevent most of this from happening throughout life. We could catch TMJoint issues and assaults on the TNS early, and take measures to balance the skeleton via the skeleton exposed in the mouth, the vertical support pillars of teeth, preventing the forward head posture from ever occurring. If this were examined for and significantly eliminated early in life, most of this pain as well as the needless surgeries and years of drugs could be avoided. The earlier in life that it's caught and treated, the better for all. If podiatrists can equalize leg length throughout life via custom orthotics in the shoes, imagine how much back pain, neck pain, knee and hip pain could be prevented by providing perfect balance and alignment throughout the entire skeleton. The body is like any other building or structure. It's going to be stronger, healthier, and more beautiful if all the support structures are equal and balanced in length. The human body is a skyscraper on two pillars that move. You don't want your head posture throwing off the whole structure. Just watch a young infant take some of its earliest steps. The weight of her head determines

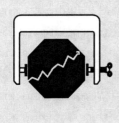

NEWSWORTHY TRUTH

HEADFIRST PREVENTIVE MEDICINE: If the skeleton of the head is examined first, rather than last or not at all, we can prevent a lifetime of unnecessary pain.

her direction, her balance and if she is going to end up on her rump. It's exaggerated in infancy, but the same thing is happening to us as adults, but to a lesser degree.

According to insurance companies, because I'm a dentist I'm not allowed to treat the trigeminal nerve using major medical codes regarding symptoms caused by the TNS. However, the TNS is the main innervation of every structure that dentists deal with daily. The state licensing board has backed us, but the insurance companies are still allowed to deny our patients the coverage for which they are paying premiums. How are major medical insurance companies permitted to receive monthly premiums and yet exclude treatment for the largest of the twelve cranial nerves, the TNS? There are laws in the state of Wisconsin that clearly state dentists are permitted to treat migraines and other symptoms as physicians or other medical specialties are permitted to treat these different symptoms, and yet insurance companies still deny their clients' claims for dental treatment. And for some reason, the office of the insurance commissioner has no power to override these companies' practices.

The other day I had to tell a patient who had severe trigeminal neuralgia that I cannot treat any structures that are supplied by the TN and expect to be paid by her insurance company for the treatment. She has three missing teeth, and her remaining teeth have shifted. The pain she is enduring daily will not go away by itself. Because of this lack of coverage, the patient chose not to go forward with the treatment. I can't blame her. I know that paying out of pocket can be a financial burden, especially when you pay for insurance that should be responsible to cover your medical needs. Instead, this patient, like so many, will continue to go from doctor to doctor wasting the insurance company's money as well as her own on treatments the insurance will cover, while getting no permanent pain relief. How ridiculous is that?

A LIFETIME OF SUFFERING AVERTED

Marilyn appeared in my office about thirty-five years ago. She sat in the reception room, exhausted and disheveled. Severe vertigo made her grip the chair for fear of falling off. She had been in Michigan with her parents and was unable to travel back home to Wisconsin in any moving vehicle because of the vertigo and headaches. A dentist in Toronto, Canada, put a large, upper splint in her mouth that managed vertigo enough so that she could travel. Finally back in Wisconsin, she went to an ophthalmologist who told her she had Ménière's disease.

Marilyn's symptoms got so bad at one point that her parents came over from Michigan to pick up her kids. Her husband planned to have her committed to an institution because she was unable to function. She had several missing teeth, dislocated TMJoints, and severe muscle spasms in the head face and neck. Even with these symptoms, no one other than the Toronto dentist who had helped her, pointed out the connection to her dental issues and her suffering. She had so many missing teeth and such badly damaged joints we had to use two different appliances to aggressively treat her case.

Once she felt better, Marilyn went back to the ophthalmologist to get new glasses. He insisted on his diagnosis of Ménière's disease and said the vertigo would be back. But if Marilyn accepted his misdiagnosis, which the ophthalmologist offered without examining her mouth or TMJoints, and not sought treatment in our office, she could have been condemned to a lifetime of vertigo, severe headaches, the loss of her two children, as well as being institutionalized!

Let's not forget: the ophthalmologist received payment for his testing and misdiagnosis by the medical insurance industry. Marilyn and her family had to pay out-of-pocket costs for the "TMJ treatment" that relieved her pain and solved her vertigo.

Imagine the cost to insurance companies and the state if she had spent the past thirty-five years in an institution? This is another example of the atrocities being perpetrated on patients all over the world while this epidemic pain for profit is permitted to spread unchecked.

We recently shot a video of Marilyn at her home for a documentary we are producing. Marilyn gave us a tour of photographs of her holding and playing with her grandchildren. She said, "I would never have been able to experience all this joy had I never found you thirty-five years ago."

THE DIFFICULT TRUTH

How likely do you think it is that the medical clinics, hospitals, pharmaceutical companies, chiropractic and osteopathic clinics in the United States are going to willingly give up these profitable patients? Could money be the reason that insurance companies refuse to cover treatment that can eliminate the pain without drugs and surgeries? After all, if the pain is eliminated, the money train for these hospitals, medical clinics, and pain clinics comes to a screeching halt.

In my opinion, what these insurance companies are doing to poor suffering people and their families is morally wrong. Even when presented with proof of improvement and progress reports signed by

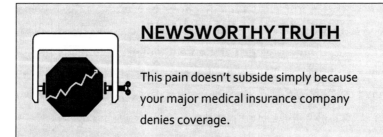

NEWSWORTHY TRUTH

This pain doesn't subside simply because your major medical insurance company denies coverage.

patients who are relieved to be living without pain and without drugs, insurance companies continue to deny coverage. Interestingly, these companies are more than willing to accept premiums and set up a team of investigators to stop the one treatment that has ended or relieved most of my clients' symptoms for the first time in decades. Can you give me one reason why a major medical insurance company would want to set up roadblocks and deny coverage for an effective treatment that could save them hundreds of billions of dollars?

A TRUTH THAT PRISONERS OF PAIN NEED TO KNOW

This treatment can free them from the prisons of:
1.   Chronic pain
2.   Endless drugs
3.   Endless medical bills
4.   Poor sleep
5.   Chronic fatigue
6.   Chronic depression
7.   Lost relationships

The sad truth is this pain doesn't subside simply because your major medical insurance company denies coverage. If you choose to do nothing and not take action, you will be condemned to a life of seeking treatments that are covered, but do not offer a cure or long-term solution. The truth is, you must make your health a priority even if your insurance company does not.

Before enduring surgery, I urge you to consult with a dentist who devotes the bulk of his/her practice (50 to 70 percent) to relieving chronic pain. Let a qualified dentist examine you to see if your pain is TMJ- or TNS-related.

Find help and healing. Then, when you are feeling healthy and whole, take things into your own hands and follow instructions in the chapter titled "Unite for the Cause" and pursue reimbursement for the treatment. I am convinced that if enough of the millions of people suffering with this pain will do this, insurance companies will be forced to cover this effective treatment in the future.

WHAT ARE DENTISTS DOING TO HELP THE ISSUE?

HERE'S THE UGLY TRUTH: THE DENTAL PROFESSION AS A WHOLE DOESN'T WANT TO CLAIM RESPONSIBILITY FOR THE TREATMENT OF CHRONIC TNS- AND TMJ-RELATED PAIN. Although we have the honor of being the only members of the medical community with the ability to cure a huge percentage of chronic pain in the world without drugs or surgery, most dentists don't want to assume this role. A number of reasons factor into this truth, not the least of which is the fact that the sheer number of patients and the severity of the pain they suffer makes the responsibility and burden of treating the ailments seem overwhelming.

Insurance Companies Refuse to Cover Treatment

In defense of my profession, I feel it's important to point out that many more dentists would be treating this by now if insurance companies didn't make it so stressful and time consuming to collect payment for services rendered, and be constantly denied. Goliath insurance companies have beaten many dentists into submission; good friends of mine have stopped treating this because they're tired of battling insurance companies.

As stated earlier, the reality is, major[31] medical insurance companies have put up roadblock after roadblock, and denial after denial, regarding dentists treating migraines and multiple symptoms related to the TNS and TMJoints. These roadblocks exist, despite the fact that medical and insurance industries have known for decades that the TNS is the primary cause of headaches and migraines. I've already explained that in its infinite wisdom, the insurance industry refuses to recognize the TMJoints as part of the human body. The insurance industry should know that everything we dentists deal with every day is innervated by the TNS, thereby making us best equipped to turn off the multiple triggers to the TNS and eliminate the symptoms. As discussed in the previous chapter, despite evidence and scientific proof that dentists can eliminate many forms of chronic pain by balancing the bite, insurance companies in many states still refuse to cover the necessary treatment. The bottom line is, if patients can't pay for the treatment and the insurance companies refuse to cover it, the dentist doesn't get paid. No one can work for free on an ongoing basis and still pay their mortgage, so many dentists stick to procedures for which they know they'll be paid.

The Responsibility is Overwhelming

The insurance debacle isn't the only reason so few dentists, relatively speaking, examine for and treat this disorder. The huge responsibility of the issue undoubtedly factors in as well. Similar to the tobacco industry not wanting to raise its hand and say its products cause cancer, dentistry doesn't want the responsibility for the enormous amount of chronic pain they can cure. Nor do they want to acknowledge the pain they can cause with less-than-perfect dental work. However, with proper training, this could become a non-issue.

Dental Schools Don't Provide Training

Unfortunately, the scarcity of proper training is also a problem. For some dentists, it isn't willful negligence or denial, but simply ignorance. Many dental schools don't teach dentists how to properly examine patients for TNS-related issues. The reason? The faculty at one dental school told me it's too complicated to teach the mechanics and technology required for this treatment, so they don't include it in the general dental curriculum. Think about that. If you've taken the self-exam included in this book, you know that some of the signs indicative of this problem are obvious. Why, then, would it be so difficult to teach how to examine for and diagnose this issue and then refer patients to qualified dentists as they already do for root canals, periodontal surgery, orthodontics, and oral surgery?

It certainly is not too complex to teach how to diagnose. Nor is it unreasonable to expect new dentists to be taught what causes this pain so they won't fabricate restorations, crowns, and removable prostheses like partials and dentures that can trigger years of this life-altering pain. The precision of treating bites with this type of balance and immediate guidance systems would be worth several lectures during the course of their four years of dental school. Understanding the three-dimensional environment of the triplane comfort position initially may be a challenge, but when dentists realize they hold the key to preventing so many chronic symptoms that afflict their patients, friends, and family members, they will become excited. It's a wonderful feeling to offer people real relief and to see the quality of their lives improve.

Over the past thirty-seven years, I've met with three different deans of my alma mater, Marquette University Dental School, and offered to lecture or help set up curriculum to help students understand, examine for, diagnose, and refer or treat patients for this problem. The hygiene department was very interested and they had me back several times, but the dental school? Never. I have offered to come speak to the dental students as a guest lecturer free of charge, and still no call. It fell on deaf ears. I can understand why other professions hate to see this come to fruition, but dentistry? The current dean and his associate met with me before the new dental school was completed, and I told him this could use its own wing. He said all space was planned, but they would be interested in my help in making it part of curriculum. The associate dean was very excited as I described the life-giving changes we are privileged to witness in our practice every week, but that too must have been quelled back at the office. No one called to involve me in the curriculum planning.

The fact that so many young dentists remain under-educated in this area frustrates me. Twenty years ago, I met with the head of admissions of a dental school when one of my sons was considering following in my footsteps. I asked if the four-year program included any training in this area of expertise. After beating around the bush, the answer was basically no. To which I responded: "So you want us to pay you over $100,000 to produce a dinosaur relative to something this important?" Unfortunately, and coincidently, this conversation happened about the same time we were bringing this problem before the legislature in Wisconsin to mandate coverage; dentists and dental associations understood the scope of this problem even then, and too many schools still refuse to address it in the general curriculum.

Dentistry's "Permission to Ignore"

Since the 1950s, a number of textbooks have been written on the subject of treatment. These textbooks and other books and articles, date back centuries to 1758, 1894, and in the case of Hippocrates all the way back to about 300 BC. They all make an obvious connection between the teeth, the bite, TMJoint dislocations, and MPD (muscle spasms), with chronic head, neck, and facial pain. (Some of these works are noted in the section of this book titled "Chronic Pain: Truths Through the Ages," beginning on page 34). These texts were written for the dental and medical professionals, and they have been ignored in exactly the same way the dental and medical professions have ignored the TNS and TMJoints in physical examinations for centuries.

For some reason, the entire dental community has been given a pass on whether or not to ask patients, "Do you suffer from any chronic pain symptoms such as headache, migraine, neck pain, eye pain, ear pain, or vertigo?" Call almost any dental office this morning with toothache pain, and they'll get you in by this afternoon. But if you call complaining about migraines that you have lived with for decades, they won't get you in for an exam, they will rarely refer you, and they won't know how to treat you. How can this go on when so much evidence points to dentistry as the one profession that can relieve patients of this pain?

Is Curriculum Influenced by Big Pharma?

Another reason I suspect factors into dental schools' resistance or neglect to teach students how to cure patients without drugs or surgery is the result of pressure put on schools by pharmaceutical companies. In *The Truth About the Drug Companies*, Marcia Angell, M.D., mentions that pharmaceutical companies have people on the boards of medical schools offering input on the curriculum.[15]

How much of the hundreds of billions of dollars of the pharmaceutical industry's annual income do you think it would take to acquire an influential position at a dental school? If these companies are acting as "benefactors" and contributing to dental schools for the privilege of influencing or even dictating portions of the curriculum, students are, in effect, being short-changed on their education. Worse, patients worldwide continue to pay to suffer every time they fill another prescription to mask the pain, but not address the cause.

DENTAL ASSOCIATIONS MUST BEGIN INSISTING ON THOROUGH EXAMS AND PROPER TREATMENT

While some new dentists may not be aware they should be watching for TNS- and TMJ-related issues, dental associations cannot claim ignorance. Dentistry has long been aware of how much this treatment helps relieve migraines, recurring headaches and many other symptoms. Professional dental associations recognize that the TNS-related pain is a major medical, neurological, orthopedic problem and should be covered by major medical insurance like any other joint and major nerve system, whether the treating doctor is a physician or dentist.

In 1997, I joined with the Wisconsin Dental Association (WDA) and helped spearhead a drive to pass a state law requiring that TMJoints be recognized as part of the body and covered by major medical insurance. It was called a TMJ bill because TMJ is a catch-all term, like Kleenex, the trademarked term now used as the generic term for tissue. For some reason it is easier for patients and those within the medical community to believe that it is not the TNS causing all this referred pain, but rather just the TMJoints. Perhaps that's true because they can see and understand how the joints operate and the TNS isn't visible. Regardless, the important truth here is that I am not alone in my belief that the TNS is a primary cause of many types of chronic pain, migraines, and tension headaches. The WDA, and other state and national associations absolutely were aware that the teeth, TNS, TMJoints, and the chewing muscles (muscles of mastication) are capable of causing pain. That's why the WDA went to Wisconsin's state capital to get the law passed that mandated that major medical insurances had to cover the TMJoints.[28] It was a step in the right direction. Now we need other associations nationwide to take this step as well.

Ten years after the Wisconsin TMJ bill was signed, a female president of the American Dental Association (ADA), only the second female ever, was asked by a reporter for *Dental Images*,[26] the Marquette

Dental School magazine, what she believed to be the biggest issues facing dentistry today. And guess what? She listed access to dental care, government funded programs, future of dental education, electronic patient records, improved oral health for the elderly, etc. Who can dispute any of these? They're always on the list of needs. But what shocked me was that she, who was present the day the Wisconsin TMJ bill was signed, never mentioned TMJ treatment or dentistry's major role in curing chronic pain. Talk about a slap in the face to the millions of women suffering across America since the bill was passed in 1997. *When millions and millions of people (three-quarters of whom are women) suffer daily with severe pain and migraines, much of which could be relieved by dentists, that suffering and the lack of attention it receives should be worth mentioning as one of the biggest issues facing dentistry today!*

I'm not naïve. I know that this past president, the WDA, and the ADA primarily represent general dentistry. But does that mean all these suffering people should continue to suffer for decades while dentistry's hierarchy decides whether they want accept their responsibility to diagnose and either learn to treat or refer patients to trained dentists? Dentistry as a whole prides itself on being very preventive compared to most health professions. Based on that alone, these groups should want to bring this problem and treatment to the forefront of modern medicine. Organized dentistry knows this problem exists. Even though dentistry has not made this a specialty area like surgery, endodontics, periodontics or orthodontia, a number of associations and academies have journals and meetings focused solely on this problem. An example would be the American Academy of Craniofacial Pain. These groups understand the problem and recognize that specially trained dentists are the only doctors in the medical community who have the technology and expertise to alter the bite to change these forces traumatizing the TNS, teeth, muscles and TMJoints. This knowledge demands that all dental associations must recognize the severity of this issue. They must insist that their members examine every patient for these problems and refer those who suffer on a frequent basis from any of these chronic pain symptoms to a qualified dentist. Until that happens patients will continue to go undiagnosed, untreated, and suffering for decades.

The good news is: change is possible. When patients, dentists, dental schools, dental associations, the medical profession, and the insurance industry get on board and make examinations, diagnosis and treatment of chronic suffering a priority—and commit to stopping the practice of pain for profit—the benefits for patients will be innumerable. How do I know change is possible? I've seen it happen in the dental world before.

THE UPSIDE OF CHANGE

In the late 1960s and early 1970s, Dr. Robert Barkley introduced the world to preventive dentistry through plaque control. Prior to Dr. Barkley, the general assumption and acceptance was that people would lose their teeth in their old age. Working with a group called the American Society of Preventive Dentistry, he introduced flossing as a means to remove plaque and prevent tooth decay and gum disease. A totally new concept at that time, his lectures and writings on the necessity of flossing and preventive dentistry swept through dentistry and changed dentistry forever. Today, because of preventative dental care and flossing, Baby Boomers have greatly reduced their risk of tooth loss in later years.

The acceptance that plaque control has received is exactly what the world needs in regard to the diagnosis and treatment of chronic pain relative to the TNS, the teeth, muscles of mastication, and the TMJoints. The message that teeth are support pillars in the skeleton of the skull, that the laws of physics apply to the body, and that the TNS can be linked to migraines and referred pain throughout the body, and most importantly, that trained dentists can reduce or eliminate many types of chronic pain by balancing the bite, must go right to the heart of dentistry and change the face of dentistry again.

If this problem were only about the dental benefits it affords the patient, it should sweep the profession. When the traumatic forces and torque exerted on teeth through an imbalanced bite are analyzed, reduced, and eliminated, it will do more for the prevention of gum disease, root canals and tooth loss than all the flossing in the world. Treating TNS- and TMJ-related problems can drastically reduce the bone loss caused by gum disease, glancing traumatic forces, chronic clenching and bruxing. Additionally, it will reduce the occurrences of fractured teeth, sensitive teeth, unnecessary root canals, and tooth loss. And those are only the benefits from a dental prospective. When you throw in the elimination of the long list of chronic pain symptoms (see page 25), the effects of this movement could be nothing short of miraculous.

I hope dentistry will pick up the gauntlet with pride and lead this health movement. But even Dr. Barkley's plaque control movement was not met with open arms by the profession or the public for that matter. I distinctly remember a patient who came to my office for a cleaning and was none too happy when I explained she had severe gum problems. Evidently, I was the first dentist to examine her gums. I explained the issue, showed her how to floss, and charged her $35 (you can guess this happened a number of years ago). She left my office and never returned. I found out later she went back to the dentist that allowed the 5-7 millimeter pockets to form without telling her. She didn't like the change I

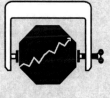

NEWSWORTHY TRUTH

When the traumatic forces and torque exerted on teeth through an imbalanced bite are analyzed, reduced, and eliminated, it will do more for the prevention of gum disease and tooth loss than all the flossing in the world.

proposed to her dental routine. Over time, flossing has become a standard accepted practice for preventative dental care.

I mentioned in an earlier chapter that Dr. Harold Gelb predicted back in 1974 that it would take twenty-five years before dental schools would teach students how to relieve patients of chronic pain. I was blessed to run into him and a number of my other mentors at a weekend symposium put on by the American Academy of Craniofacial Pain, in Indianapolis in September of 2008. I told him I was sad to report that he was wrong on his projection. He said, "I know, you have to add another twenty-five years on top of that."

As Columbus told his son in the opening scene of the movie Columbus, "Change is rarely met with unanimous acceptance." They had just watched a ship disappear over the horizon, and Columbus asked his son if he thought the world was flat and the ship dropped off the edge. He then held up an orange and rotated it keeping his finger in one spot. His finger disappeared to the other side of the orange, out of sight.

We no longer view the world as flat. We have documented proof that it is indeed round. Similarly, the dental profession has access to a wealth of books and articles that have been written over the centuries connecting the teeth to headaches and neck pain. It is just as ignorant to say the world is flat as it is to continue viewing the bite as a separate entity that has no effect on the skeleton of the head and neck.

With improved technology and adequate knowledge, it is possible to change the way we treat chronic pain. For that to happen, however, the

---

It is just as ignorant to say the world is flat as it is to continue viewing the bite as a separate entity that has no effect on the skeleton of the head and neck.

---

medical and dentistry professions must be forced out of the dark ages. They must stop ignoring history and the power of today's technology that offer visible, measurable evidence. To the dentists reading this book I offer this note: Take advantage of the technology that is available to you. I promise, you'll learn more about pathologic torque and poorly functioning guidance systems in one week on the Tekscan bite computer than you did in four years of dental school.

EDUCATING PATIENTS, FORCING CHANGE

It's important to me that dentists know I've tried conventional ways to change the laws and accepted practices regarding TNS- and TMJ-related pain to literally no avail. Going through accepted channels hasn't stopped the epidemic or the practice of pain for profit. But I'm sixty-seven years old and being "nice" and playing by the rules isn't working fast enough for me to get this message out. A few years ago, I realized that unless I embarked on a mission to educate chronic pain sufferers themselves to take action, nothing was going to change.

I started treating patients for migraines and chronic pain in September of 1974. Nine years later, I was certain I was onto something very big. Even at that time, with limited understanding and technology, I had an extremely high success rate for relieving chronic pain symptoms and migraines.

In 1983, I appeared before the legislative committee of the Wisconsin Dental Association. I was already so passionate about the change I was seeing in these patients' lives; my colleagues didn't seem to share my enthusiasm. After speaking on the subject for thirty minutes, I distinctly remember finishing with a lump in my throat, saying, "I can tell by the look on your faces that you all think this is an option for dentistry, whether to diagnose or treat this problem, or not." Twenty-six years later, the association is still not speaking forcefully enough in industry journals to make dentists believe that diagnosing this problem is not an option.

A Note to Dentists

Before the shock waves of needed change are over dentists need to take courses to cover themselves and learn how to be part of the most fulfilling area of dentistry.

Have you ever walked into a store, had a patient grab you and introduce you to her elderly mother saying, "Mom I want you to meet my savior! He's the one who got rid of all that pain!" I have. I've also been called a "miracle worker" and a "freakin' genius." Perhaps most touching was the patient who told me, "Because I met you thirty-five years ago, I'm here today. My kids would have been taken away from me, I'd have been placed in a mental institution, and I would never have played with my grandchildren... I'd be dead by now."

Just as you can, I have learned a skill that enables me to cure patients of their chronic pain symptoms. As an individual dentist you have the right to choose not to treat, but as more and more patients learn to examine themselves for TMJ- and TNS-related pain, you can expect to refer a large number of your patients out of your practice to be treated by someone else if you don't learn how to treat this fulfilling area of dentistry. Dentists who choose not to treat are not only missing a big boat, they are missing a luxury liner. You could be treating and freeing all these patients that medicine has been imprisoning in pain and debt for centuries. Why wouldn't every dentist want to join the army of dentists freeing these patients from the prison of pain, and experience the joy of these miracles themselves?

For Dentists:
A Quick Summary of Obvious Signs to Examine

Regardless of whether you want to learn how to treat this problem, you must learn how to examine and diagnose patients for it. The following notes briefly explain how to examine your patients for TMJ disorders. I recommend you read the self-exam with the explanations of how each sign is a tip-off to chronic pain.

First, look for the following:

- Flattening of the pointed cusp tip on the upper and lower cuspids

- Flattening or jagged rough edges on the upper and lower front teeth

- Lack of immediate lateral and protrusive anterior guidance

- Facial asymmetry (one eye open more, one eyebrow higher, smile favoring one side, and the corner of one side of the mouth is higher, or one side droops more)

- Forward or lateral head posture

- One shoulder more rounded and lower than the other

- Wear facets or breaking off of posterior teeth (large over carved silver or composite restorations, crowns, and possibly multiple root canals from chasing sensitive teeth due to this problem)

- Crowded teeth or rotated teeth

- Cross bites: Unilateral, bilateral, or just one or two individual teeth in the anterior or posterior of the mouth

- Deep overbites

- Class III prognathic bites (less-frequent cause of chronic pain)

- Class II with deep overbites and retruded lower jaws are more prevalent in the arena of chronic pain

- Lack of posterior support due to broken down teeth, missing teeth, collapsing of the arch due to tooth loss without timely replacement

- Creases or wrinkles in the corners of the mouth due to over-closed bite, deep overbite and loss of vertical dimension in the bite

Next, conduct each of the following exams.

I. The Stethoscope Exam

1. Listen with a stethoscope for a clicking or popping in the joint while opening or closing to maximum opening and closure. This most often indicates that the disc is dislocated and is popping in and out during opening and closing; it reveals that the disc is not in place to provide a cushion between the bone of the condyle and the base of the skull whenever the mouth is closed.

2. Listen for grating or crepitus sounds when the patient opens or closes his mouth to maximum opening and closure. This indicates that the disc is either perforated or permanently dislocated and the bones are rubbing against each other. The rubbing is like a pharmacist's mortar and pestle, or a pool cue being chalked, damaging the bone and grinding against the auriculotemporal branch of the TNS.

3. If no stethoscope is available you can feel a high percentage of these clicks, or crepitus by placing your fingers lightly over both TMJoints as the patient opens and closes to maximum opening and closure, or by lightly cradling the mandibular bone during this opening and closing.

II. The Millimeter Ruler Exam

1. Measure the patient's overbite, the distance the upper centrals overlap the lower central incisors in a vertical direction. If this distance is more than 1.5 to 2.5 millimeters, the possibility of chronic pain increases.

2. Measure the patient's overjet, the distance the upper central incisors project in a horizontal direction in front, or the facial surface of the lower incisors. Ideally they should contact mildly to enable immediate protrusive guidance and lift off in the posterior of the mouth. If a patient has to travel 1 to 3 millimeters or more before the lower incisors engage the lingual of the upper incisors, or they never engage (open or end-to-end bite; no overjet), the opportunity for posterior interferences and the need to grind teeth and brux teeth increases. This increases the likelihood of perpetuated decades of irritation to the TN, and chronic daily pain.

3. Measure the maximum opening of the mouth from the incisal edge of the upper central incisor to the incisal edge of the lower central incisor, and add in the measurement of the patient's overbite. This is their maximum opening. You may want to place a tooth pick between the upper and lower front teeth and note whether the lower jaw deviates right, left, or both, during the maximum opening cycle, and measure the deviation. Note the deviation in the patient's record. It is indicative of dislocations in the TMJ, and whether they are closed lock or there is still reduction of the disc (a click or pop in the joint indicating the disc is reducing back into place temporarily when open). Whether closed lock or the disc is reducing on opening, the disc is still not

cushioning the joint when the patient is closed, eating, or while clenching and grinding. The possibility of pain is greatly enhanced with dislocation because the trigeminal nerve is being assaulted in the posterior aspect of the TMJoint any time the patient is closed, clenched, or grinding their teeth. In essence the TN is being ground up like a pharmacist's mortar and pestle (condyle in fossa) while the patient grinds and clenches his teeth all night long during sleep, while eating, or during stressful times during the day.

4. Measure the patient's ability to move the lower jaw to the right and the left. The lower jaw should be able to move 9 to 13 millimeters to each side. Measure off of midline of the upper centrals, and be sure to take into account how far the midline of the lower arch is off-center relative to the upper arch first.

III. The Palpation Exam (use index or little finger)

1. First palpate the TMJoints by standing behind the patient and placing the tip of your little finger into their ears and forcing it in and forward as they open wide. Give them this instruction first before placing fingers in their ears: "After you open wide and my fingers are in your ears close very slowly and see if it is even possible for you to close completely on your back molars. This may hurt a great deal, in which case do not close any further." We will know from that if the TN is being compressed due to the substantial amount of swelling and inflammation in the TMJoint in the posterior region. This is a very good indicator of TN overload, and chronic pain possibilities.

2. Apply pressure from the side of the face over the TMJoints as the patient repeats the previous instructions. If the joints are swollen and inflamed laterally it will not be comfortable to open and close with pressure applied here.

3. Use your index or middle finger to palpate the muscles of mastication, and muscles of the neck, back, and shoulders while you have the patient grade the pain and discomfort in these muscles on a scale of 0-5.

0 = no pain
1 = tender
2 = uncomfortable

3 = pain, "It hurts."
4 = hurts, "DO NOT push on that again."
5 = severe pain, "Push on it again and I'll kill you."

Have them grade each of the following muscle groups as you palpate them:

- Apply approximately two pounds of pressure on the lateral ptery-goid muscles by pushing up and inward in the area between the cheek and the upper second molars, and have them grade it zero to five. This is often extremely painful (4-5 range) because this muscle is in constant spasm trying to hold the condyle forward to decrease compression in the back of the TMJoint.

- Press on the medial pterygoid muscle in the same manner by applying pressure to the muscles at the side walls of the entrance to the throat. This is one of the clenching muscles and is often painful (4-5 range).

- Press on the superficial and deep belly of the masseter muscle by pressing on the cheek and around the back angle of the mandible for the deep belly. The masseter is the strongest muscle in the body and it's a clenching muscle. With clenchers and bruxers it is often over developed and rock hard. The deep belly toward the back angle of the mandible is generally more painful to palpation.

- Palpate the huge fan-shaped muscle over the temple areas of the head called the temporalis muscle. This is where many of these patients experience their horrendous headaches. It too, is a clenching muscle, and you should have the patient clench and relax as you palpate the muscle. The anterior belly is generally the most painful to palpation.

- Palpate the SCM (sternocleidomastoid muscles) in the neck.

- Palpate the trapezius muscles in the back of the neck. These are often graded (4-5 range) as extremely painful to palpation if the patient has already developed the forward head posture. If the head posture is forward and lateral, the trapezius muscle of the opposite side of the head is usually more painful to palpation because it is supporting more of the weight of the head.

- Palpate the occipital muscles and the base of the skull in the back of the head. This is where many of these muscles attach to the base of the skull. These muscles can be very sore when forward head posture requires them to support more of the weight of the head and its constant battle with gravity.

- Palpate the trapezius muscles from the base of the neck laterally to the top of the shoulders. These are the muscles everybody likes rubbed when getting a massage. These muscles are also working overtime with patients with the forward and lateral head posture, and they strongly interact with the deltoids causing quite severe shoulder pain in many of these patients.

- Palpate the deltoid muscles in the shoulder.

- Palpate and apply pressure to the muscles of the upper, mid, and lower back. The head weighs ten to sixteen pounds, as much as a bowling ball. With forward head and lateral head posture the muscles and weight-bearing joints all the way down the entire body are compensating and adjusting to support the off-balance weight of the head, causing pain in many strained areas of the body's muscular system, and in joints that are not functioning in a centered position.

IV. The Bite Exam

Articulating paper and Shimstock (Silver strip 1/5000th millimeters thick) are required, or more preferable, a Tekscan bite computer to check for bite imbalances and cross arch balancing interferences. Articulating paper doesn't give good readings in the area of the twelve-year molars due to saliva, and that molar is important to check for balancing interferences. It's a critical area to test for in chronic headache patients. One of the many benefits of the Tekscan bite computer is that it still gets great readings in the back of the mouth, even with saliva.

I fully realize in this economy dentists are not looking to buy new equipment, but Tekscan bite computers should be a must in every general dentistry office and in every dental specialty office. They easily pay for themselves in months if you charge for the service, which you must. *Articulating paper is archaic compared to the computer readings.* It gives no idea of the intensity of the forces, the deflective trajectory of the forces, the percent of force on each tooth, the immediacy of anterior guidance, or posterior clearance on the balancing side. The latest version of the Tekscan software and hardware is amazingly accurate. There is a slight learning curve, but for the younger generation of dentists that are already computer savvy it should be a piece of cake. It will give you an understanding of your wonderful profession you never dreamed possible: fulfillment, saving people's lives, and filling your chair all at the same time.

You are blessed to be involved in the only profession trained to treat this unique area of the body, the only place the skeleton comes through the skin. We can change it permanently without cutting the patient open with surgery, and better, we can prove the treatment works before doing anything permanent, with a diagnostic orthotic balanced with a triplane guidance system. Dentists, please get excited and, better yet, get involved, as Harold Gelb said in the first lecture I ever heard, "You are in the best profession to

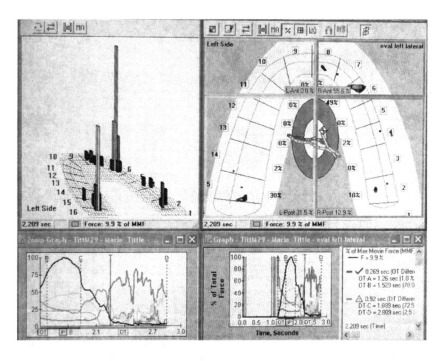

These Tekscan images illustrate the interference on the 12 year molar tooth number 15 when the patient moved jaw to the right. It should ride up on number 6 only. As explained earlier, this is a huge cause of headaches.

Become Part of the Solution!

I believe that with the vivid understanding the Tekscan computer enables us to visualize on a computer screen for the first time in the history of dentistry, most dentists could learn to enjoy these miracles in their practice. We have developed a systematic, simplistic approach to locating the triplane comfort position, "the Happy Place" (the place where pain disappears) by utilizing the bite computer to design immediate guidance systems. Most dentists would be able to easily learn how to examine and diagnose TMJ and TNS disorders. With further instruction they can learn to treat this in their practice and become part of the solution.

This pandemic is so large that it is going to take an army of dentists across the world to treat and free billions from chronic pain. Remember: This new era of Headfirst Preventive Medicine uniquely positions dentists to end chronic suffering. Feel the pride and fulfillment of being part of a miracle and part of the solution! This is your chance to help change health care in this country and around the world. My next book will offer detailed instruction for dentists on how to treat both Phase One and Two.

I hope by now you understand my passion for helping suffering people. You'll be reborn too, with your new understanding of how vital your work is to humanity.

The outlook for dentistry in the future of medicine it is very exciting. Dentistry will no longer be able to deny this to the public because the public is going to be able to survey and examine themselves. For dentistry this can be the Titanic, a luxury liner that will definitely raise dentistry's position with the public and the medical hierarchy, or it can be the iceberg that sunk the ship. What organized dentistry does with this is no longer your only option. As an individual dentist you can join the cause and be part of the solution!

help people who are suffering from chronic pain." In addition to that you get to develop great relationships with these wonderful people and their families as you witness the miracle of the rebirth of an adult free of pain; and if you're really lucky, you'll get to see the wonderful effect it has on their children and spouse as well. Don't miss out. Are there bumps in the road? Yes. But nothing compared to the miracles that you get to orchestrate because of your knowledge.

V. Periodic Recall Evaluation for Dental Patients

Ask: Are you suffering from headaches, neck, ear, facial pain or vertigo (or dizziness) with any regularity since last exam?

Ask: Are any teeth particularly sensitive since last visit? Keep articulating red and blue paper handy to quickly evaluate and set up necessary equilibration to fine-tune bite and avoid fractures and needless root canals.

Look: Has the patient fractured off any teeth since last evaluation? Look especially at molars or guidance teeth in the anterior.

Look: Is there any increase in pocket depths anywhere in the mouth? This can be a tip-off to traumatic occlusion. Have red and blue articulating paper available in these instances. Set up an appointment to equilibrate these areas once every two years, with a Tekscan computer if possible, and you'll watch gum disease disappear in your practice. Dentistry has taken the lead on prevention of dental disease with plaque control via flossing, brushing and fluoride treatments. Monitoring and equilibrating and equalizing pressure and torque throughout the bite will literally stop most gum disease, fractures, root canals, and tooth loss.

I know it sounds as though this treatment will put us out of business; it won't. Millions in the USA, and billions worldwide, suffer from chronic pain, dislocated TMJoints and neuromuscular spasms. They need our help. Treating patients and relieving them of this constant suffering is completely fulfilling; it is life changing because it gives your patients a better quality of life. And isn't that why you went into dentistry in the first place?

A WORD ON TECHNOLOGY

Today we have technologies like the Tekscan bite computer that lets us literally see the intensity of forces, the timing of forces, the immediacy of guidance, and the lack of contact and support when patients are amputees of the skeleton of the skull or their support pillars (teeth) are broken down to a point that they don't contact. The Tekscan computer display is almost like the Disney movie Fantasia. Dentists can watch colored vertical towers of forces dancing up and down while the patient's teeth collide, or *attempt* to glide, through needed chewing and grinding movements. You literally watch force and timing movies as different movements are carried out. In this era, no dentist or dental specialist on the planet should be allowed to practice without a bite computer. It should be as basic as the mirror, the explorer and periodontal probe. It offers a visual demonstration of what dentists have wanted to create since G. V. Black (1836-1915) "the father of modern dentistry" tried to use photo film in an attempt to accomplish something similar over a century ago. (Have you noticed how often that word century has been cropping up in this book? The "Good Ones" have known there's a connection between a patient's pain and his bite for a very long time.)

Now that we can actually see visual data and timing, we can orchestrate the proper balance, sequencing, and timing of contact and guidance systems to appease the TNS, muscles, bones, teeth, and dislocated joints on many fronts. Dentistry as a whole thinks this technology is unnecessary. The entire modern world uses computerized technology; why does dentistry think technology is optional? They use technology when it comes to aesthetics, straightening and teeth whitening. Why would facial symmetry and eliminating chronic pain be any less important?

I have had several upgrades of this computer system since 1992. Not once in those past 20 years has a patient come into my practice and said, "My dentist has one of those." This must change. Do you have to have a Tekscan or similar system to treat this? No, but it will speed up your education and understanding. This technology also helps you achieve better results because it picks up and gives you information far beyond the red and blue articulating papers dentists have used for years. This bite computer will give every dentist and every dental specialist an understanding of the unique pathological engineering that takes place in all the different varieties of normal, dislocated and malfunctioning bites that are in total disarray. In my opinion, no dentist, orthodontist, periodontist, endodontist, oral surgeon, or maxillofacial surgeon should practice without it.

The Tekscan is the primary tool in development of this new field of Headfirst Preventive Medicine. Using it will give you the necessary understanding of the function of the bite in all the different movements, as well as the triplane comfort position. Once you learn how to use it, you will feel very confident about proceeding with the permanent alterations to the teeth that will restore the needed vertical height and guidance systems to provide the decompression of the TMJoints and eliminate the assaults on the TNS, providing the Phase Two, long-term cure.

In addition to helping the dentist and the patient see exactly what is causing the unbalanced bite and resulting pain, it also saves data that can then be referred to during treatment or for legal back up. On its own it will prevent the loss of teeth due to needless root canals and gum disease that develop when certain teeth receive abnormal amounts of torque and stress. In my follow up, how-to book for dentists, I'll include instruction on how to use this technology. In the meantime, I recommend that you look into the Tekscan technology at Tekscan.com and give your dental practice, your patients, and yourself a revolutionary gift that will change the way you see dentistry from here forward.

Dentists have a Responsibility to Stop the Pain-for-Profit Cycle

In 1959, Nathan Shore, DDS, published his first edition of *Temporomandibular Joint Dysfunction and Occlusal Equilibration*. On the opening page of the text he quotes Hippocrates, "Divine is the work to relieve pain." I am in total agreement with Shore's statement. I cannot stand by and let those in my profession miss the most rewarding and fulfilling area of dentistry. And I certainly cannot allow millions and billions of people to live as prisoners of pain in dungeons of darkness because no one is being held responsible for examining these obvious structures... yet.

This chronic pain issue can be viewed by those in dentistry as the opportunity of a lifetime in these horrible economic times. Or, it can be avoided like the plague—seen as a source of worry because of the added responsibility it places on the profession as a whole.

Will diagnosing and either referring patients to qualified dentists for treatment or addressing the issue themselves change the way they practice and perform dentistry? Yes!

Will improved education in the area enable them to understand dentistry better? Yes! Will their careers be more fulfilling all around? Completely!

Will the ability to help relieve patients of chronic pain raise their self-esteem as well as respect for the entire profession in the hierarchy of the medical profession as a whole? Absolutely! Especially respect by the public after all the bugs and less-precise technologies are purged from the profession. Dentistry will become an admired profession for its precision and ability to give people back their lives. And with 4.5 billion people worldwide suffering from headaches, according to the World Health Organization[24], not to mention the countless others who suffer from all manner of chronic pain issues caused by the TNS, teeth, TMJoints, and chewing and clenching muscles, there are plenty of people who need the help of well-trained dentists.

My prayer is that this book will help free dental schools to train dentists to treat suffering patients. If I were a new graduate of a dental school and had paid hundreds of thousands of dollars for my education, I would expect a very thorough education—an education that would have included training on how to cure this very common problem. If I paid that kind of money and was involved in a lawsuit for not recognizing a treatable condition or, worse, exacerbating it, I would question the value of my education and the integrity of the school. To be clear, I'm not saying it is necessary for every dentist to learn how to treat TNS- and TMJ-related pain. Dentists must, however, be taught how to examine and diagnose patients with this issue so they can refer them to a specialist for treatment. Dentists must be forced to at least know enough about this problem to examine and diagnose to inform patients and give them the option to seek help. This is very important; they need to know enough about this so at the very least, they don't cause it.

Just as there are dentists who specialize in orthodontics or oral surgery, many dentists, when equipped with the necessary training, will be more than happy to take on the highly technical demands and risks involved with this field. I, for one, find this specialty to be immensely rewarding. In what other areas of their practice do dentists get to change lives and see miracles every day?

The need for well-trained dentists is huge. And while there are many dentists who currently treat the cause of this pain, when millions of sufferers across the nation finally understand the source of their pain and realize they have the opportunity to be free of it, there will not be nearly enough dentists available to treat them. The world needs dentists who will step up and commit to helping people not only have healthy teeth and gums, but *pain-free* lives as well. Yes, there is learning a curve and a responsibility to continually educate and equip ourselves with the most up-to-date technology and treatments available. But as with any subject, ignorance can be overcome with knowledge. **If your state or national dental association would like to have me speak about this treatment, contact my office at 414-961-2484 or send an email to help@stoptheheadache.com.**

There will be a follow-up book for dentists and other medical professionals on how to diagnose and treat TMJ-related pain. But first, doctors and dentists must be forced to look.

PART III

HOPE FOR
CHRONIC PAIN SUFFERERS

UNITE FOR THE CAUSE:
HELP END CHRONIC PAIN
AND SUFFERING

"I was in constant pain, so things were difficult at work and at home. I'm a railroad engineer and couldn't miss work, so I simply had to work in pain. I spent several thousand dollars seeking an answer. I saw three orthopedic specialists, had twenty-five chiropractic appointments and over thirty physical therapy appointments with no relief. Then I went to a neurologist who found the herniated disc on an MRI. He had set up surgery to fuse C-5 and C-6 vertebrae the following Monday. Someone at the physical therapy office told me not to have the neck fusion until I saw Dr. Seymour at The Chronic Pain Solution Center.

Dr. Seymour convinced me to postpone surgery for a month and a half. At the time, I couldn't raise my arm to brush my hair or my teeth without severe pain. Within two months with Dr. Seymour, I was back playing on two softball teams, and swimming 500 yards a day, and I didn't have to have the surgery."

—Fred, former chronic pain sufferer

MY MISSION IS TO EDUCATE AND OPEN THE EYES OF THE PEOPLE WHO ARE ENDURING ALL THIS NEEDLESS SUFFERING AROUND THE WORLD. This book contains the truths and the knowledge needed to confront physicians, specialists, sub-specialists, administrators, and medical insurance carriers. These individuals and conglomerates should be forced to explain why they have allowed patients to lose years of their lives to pain. It certainly isn't because treatment isn't available. Large cities typically have a number of specially-trained dentists to which patients can be referred. No, treatment is definitely available in large cities, but those profiting from pain do not want to lose money by referring patients out of their network. If that isn't abuse of your rights as a patient, I don't know what is.

The money tree that is growing at the expense of chronic pain sufferers must be stopped, and stopped now! The medical community will only be forced to read this book and change their way of examining patients if you and I and millions of other chronic pain sufferers hold them accountable.

We are going to need patients with the means and courage to challenge the insurance companies, doctors, and dentists who have been permitted to ignore the TNS, the strongest muscles in the body, the TMJ, and the obvious misalignment of teeth, missing, fractured and worn teeth that contribute to chronic pain.

How do we unite and stop this epidemic of pain and the injustice of pain for profit that affects predominantly women and the elderly? Chronic pain sufferers and their friends and family members—you—can play a critical role in forcing health professionals and insurance companies to acknowledge the truth that the TNS and TMJoints are a major cause of headaches, neck pain, and numerous other chronic pain symptoms. The billions of sufferers worldwide need to make themselves heard, starting with the millions right here in the United States.

To succeed in bringing the necessary attention to this issue, we need to make a coordinated effort. There is strength in truth, and there is strength in numbers, but if we all strike out on our own, our presence won't be organized, and it won't be felt. The Internet is the vehicle that will make it possible to spread these truths and share information. I've said repeatedly that I hope you will tell everyone you know who suffers from migraines, tension headaches, neck and shoulder pain and other chronic pain symptoms. But don't stop there. To affect change we're going to have to inundate this broken system and demand change. Below are a few ways you can help.

1. SEND LETTERS AND EMAILS TO THE HEALTH PROFESSIONALS WHO HAVE KEPT YOU IN PAIN ALL THESE YEARS.

Contact the people who have kept you suffering by not examining you or not explaining the treatment options. Doctors and dentists who don't examine, diagnose, or refer patients with these symptoms need to be confronted. If you've done the self-exam and your symptoms are obvious, wouldn't it make sense that a medical professional should have, at a minimum, performed the same exam? This is either a matter of integrity or ignorance. Doctors and dentists must be held responsible for willful negligence. And if for some inexplicable reason these professionals are uninformed about the connection between the TNS and TMJoints and chronic pain, for heaven's sake, give them a copy of this book. But first, meet with them and confront them with the very obvious truths listed in the book. Ask them if you have any rights in this situation. And if your treatment for TMJoint therapy or the TNS is not covered by your insurance you might ask if they would be willing to give back some of the money you've paid them over the years and decades to help cover the treatment you need to address the cause properly. It will get the doctors and the administrators of these clinics thinking about this, and the risk management division of the malpractice insurance companies as well.

2. PURSUE YOUR INSURANCE COMPANY FOR COVERAGE AND/OR REIMBURSEMENT FOR TREATMENT.

This is precisely why I believe women are going to have to start a new "Suffer-age Movement" demanding their medical rights. In the 2012 movie "Lincoln," there's a scene in which every man in congress stands in outrage at the mention of women receiving the right to vote. In the world of medicine today it seems that many are standing in opposition to women receiving this cure. Doctors keep blaming you and your inability to cope or hormones, and their treatment in most cases is more drugs or surgery.

The elderly are going to have to do the same, or better yet join in with the women's movement. Medicine, the pharmaceutical industry, and dentistry will all require this movement to make this change happen, but the managers at major medical insurance companies are the bullies that every patient encounters when they find out they have this problem, and the insurance carriers are allowed to just sit there and deny claims time and time again. You're paying for coverage on all joints and nerves in the body, and they are denying you the right to have the treatment that will end years of your pain and suffering. Refuse to allow this any longer!

Further on in this chapter I will explain how we will help to organize and coordinate this movement. I've said it before: It makes absolutely no sense that these companies can get away with not covering what is perhaps the most vital joint in the entire body. It is irresponsible that they neglect to cover the cost of treatment for an area of the body that affects so many aspects of your life and well being. Don't stop with the outsourced person who answers the phone in the customer service center. Be relentless in getting your claims reviewed. One letter probably won't be enough when it comes to your insurance company. They are as adept at ignoring clients as they are at denying claims. Each and every insurance company needs to be inundated with letters from their clients demanding their coverage. Insurance companies need to know they are under assault. Have your company call and ask why they are paying all this money for health insurance coverage and it doesn't cover a joint and nerve that are vital to your existence, and would save them thousands of dollars in sick days. Those of you who have the means should consult an attorney and ask if you have any rights in this situation. It won't take many legal victories to change this for everyone.

3. CONTACT POLITICAL LEADERS WHO CAN HELP CHANGE THE LAWS.

Help us inundate the Department of Health and Human Services in the President's Cabinet, your state and national congressman, and state insurance commissioners with the message that the laws regarding insurance coverage must be changed. This is a very serious money game for the insurance and pharmaceutical companies. It is unlikely that they will change their policies unless the laws force them to. Don't make this harder than it needs to be. You can send basically the same letter or email to all these different departments and congressman. They need to know that huge masses of women voters and elderly are very upset.

If you have time, get involved by volunteering to help us coordinate this effort, make phone calls to political leaders, and send and answer emails and letters. Please let us know if you can help at help@stoptheheadache.com.

4. CONTACT INTERNATIONAL, NATIONAL, STATE, AND LOCAL DENTAL AND MEDICAL GROUPS.

Let these medical and dental groups know that their doctors will be confronted with these truths and asked why their professions have allowed patients to suffer all these years. They need to know this "Suffer-age Movement" is demanding to be heard. Again, you can send basically the same letter to these groups with some minor alterations. Medical and dental societies must educate the physicians and dentists who look to them for guidance. By making chronic pain treatment a priority and requiring their members to examine and diagnose TNS- and TMJ-related symptoms, these groups can help ensure that patients get the care they deserve. These groups should also promote patient education efforts so that every chronic pain and migraine sufferer understands how these specific areas of the body cause both local and referred pain. This may seem like a dream now, but when you make your presence felt, affordable treatment can be a reality! The truth is, these medical and dental associations will need to protect themselves—so they will educate the public.

5. *HELP BY SHARING YOUR STORY.*

Women and the elderly need to share their stories of chronic suffering with the media. To help make the most impact, send your story to help@stoptheheadache.com or connect with us through the website, stoptheheadache.com. **We want to show the media the massive numbers of people who suffer unnecessarily with migraines and chronic pain.** If we act as an organized group, we are more likely to be heard and taken seriously when we contact *Dateline, Dr. Phil, The Doctors, Dr. Oz, 60 Minutes, 20/20,* Oprah's OWN Network and *O Magazine, Ellen, Prevention Magazine, Woman's Day,* AARP, and other local, state or national media or groups whose audiences consist primarily of women and the elderly.

In your story, tell us how many years you suffered while no one in the medical or dental community ever examined you or explained that your jaw joint was dislocated. Share how angry or disappointed you felt when you were told that your insurance company doesn't have to cover the cause of your pain.

If you have connections or know people that have media connections that would enable us to get on these shows, or printed in these magazines, please contact us at help@stoptheheadache.com or 414-961-2484. If you have a story to share but don't know who to contact, email us. We will help you connect with the media and law makers. We need major media outlets to help spread the word. When the general public understands that so many types of chronic pain and headaches are caused by something that is treatable—curable—but doctors, dentists, insurance and pharmaceutical companies are earning billions by keeping people in pain... there will be a reckoning. Your personal story can bring these truths to light, and be part of changing the world.

In your letter or email, explain and share:

- The pain you have endured,

- How many years you have suffered,

- The effect this disorder has had on your relationship with your spouse, children, parents, and employers,

- How difficult it was or has been to miss out on all the things you once enjoyed or you wanted to do,

- How many doctors, pain clinics, medical clinics, chiropractors, osteopaths, acupuncturists, and psychiatric professionals you have visited in search of a cure,

- The types of drugs, procedures, tests, and surgeries you have undergone,

- The total cost of your chronic pain related visits, prescriptions, treatment and surgeries over the years.

Let them know that until you read *Stop the Headache* and finally found a dentist who focused on chronic pain and migraine relief, no doctor or dentist even looked at your mouth or jaw joints or performed the simple steps included in the self-exam. It only takes thirty seconds for a doctor to look in a patient's mouth for the most obvious signs of these disorders, and yet most doctors neglect to take even this simple, essential step. That neglect keeps patients like you in a prison of pain, a prison of drugs, and the debtor's prison of endless medical and drug bills for years.

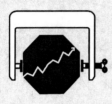

NEWSWORTHY TRUTH

It only takes thirty seconds for a doctor to look in a patient's mouth for the most obvious signs of these disorders. Most doctors neglect to take even this simple, essential step. That neglect keeps patients like you in a prison of pain, a prison of drugs, and the debtor's prison of endless medical and drug bills for years. **Sharing your story can help stop this practice of pain for profit.**

It's time to force the issue publicly. It's time to ask why, when there is an epidemic/pandemic of chronic pain that effects billions of women, elderly and poor people around the world, do patients have to learn how examine and diagnose themselves?

We need media leaders to publicly voice these questions:

- Why are doctors being permitted not to look at these structures in the skeleton and nervous system of the head and neck while this pain-for-profit industry brings in hundreds of billions of dollars each and every year?

- Why doesn't medical insurance cover a vital part of the body that is used in chewing, swallowing, digestion, speaking, sleeping, breathing and intimacy, to name just a few?

6. HELP US AMASS MASSIVE AMOUNTS OF PROOF.

Each time you send a letter or email to a political leader, dental or medical association, insurance company, physician, or media group, I ask that you send a copy of your communication to our offices at help@stoptheheadache.com. Feel free to delete or black out any account numbers, but please include your contact information.

My desire is to create a central hub of information where we can track and direct the pressure to certain key politicians, physicians, dentists, and insurance companies being called on to change their policies. This absolutely has to be a coordinated effort, and everyone is going to have to make his or her presence felt or the epidemic will continue for centuries to come.

MAKE YOUR VOICE HEARD

If you know any influential people such as politicians, corporate or religious leaders, or media personalities that would be willing to help, please send us that information as well, and have them contact us or ask if it's okay if we contact them. We need an army of people who will rally around this cause and demand that the practice of pain for profit stops. Imagine millions of letters, phone calls, and emails, sent and heard all over the medical, political, and media world. For the first time in history, social media and the Internet make it possible to get this information out to the suffering people who need hope and healing. Get excited and make your presence and your valuable story and information known!

Making this treatment available to suffering patients will lower healthcare costs *tremendously* over time, but that won't happen unless the number of people who make their voices heard is so great that these issues become impossible to ignore. Political officials must get the message that a huge voting block of suffering women, elderly, and their families and friends demand that these ridiculous insurance policies change.

WOMEN: If you are a member of a women's group, enlist the group's support in this cause. Three times as many women as men suffer from chronic pain, tension headaches, migraines and fibromyalgia. For centuries, your suffering has been ignored while you've been financially exploited. Use the clout of your women's organizations to stop this practice of pain for profit and to educate women that a cure exists. If you are the head of a women's group, or a member of a women's group or elderly group that would like to get involved in stopping this please contact us at help@stoptheheadache.com.

ELDERLY: Millions of you in the United States are dental amputees (you have missing teeth that have been extracted and not properly replaced) of the skull. As result, each year elderly patients undergo operations due to the poor head and shoulder posture—and the chronic pain that accompanies this poor posture. And millions of you know the frustration of surgeries that didn't work and the side effects of taking more and more drugs to manage recurring pain.

The entire medical field is permitted not to look at or address the structures that cause your pain. It's time for this to stop. It isn't too late for you to find relief. Make your voice heard by writing to AARP and other organized groups. Tell your story of suffering. Ask why treatment is not covered. Demand to know why the medical and dental industries have been allowed to ignore the cause of your symptoms and to keep you ignorant of a potential surgery-free and drug-free cure. As a group, those of us over age fifty-five have a lot of clout.

WE NEED AN ARMY

The world needs to understand that this problem isn't just an American issue; it is a pandemic. Women, the elderly, and the poor suffer in extraordinary numbers. It is going to require extraordinary numbers of people banning together to change the system. When we organized the campaign that got the TMJ insurance-coverage law passed in Wisconsin, we didn't just have patients call and write their congressmen. Family members, friends and coworkers who had witnessed the suffering and rebirth of cured patients also contacted these officials. That's why I say we need an army—not just of patients, but also of loved ones, caregivers, concerned citizens, attorneys, and dental professionals who treat patients for this problem. We also need medical professionals who have seen this treatment give patients back their lives and who want to help others to have medical coverage for this care. I know there are men and women — especially female physicians, nurses, dentists, etc.—who know how the current system abuses patients, particularly women. These patients need you to stand up and be heard on their behalf.

As our efforts progress, we will definitely need funding for additional studies as well as for legal counsel to set up a foundation for donations to fight the Goliaths of the "System." We will also need volunteers to handle phones, record and respond to emails, Facebook, Twitter, Blogs, and snail mail. A pain-for-profit empire of this magnitude is not going to change without all of us working together. With massive numbers of people contacting media sources, there should be so many great stories producers will want to have on their shows. When that happens, the word will get to millions of others who are suffering. My prayer is that every suffering person takes the self-exam and online survey as outlined in this book and that they will seek help with a qualified dentist if the TNS and TMJoints are the cause of their pain. I also want every doctor and administrator to know that they are no longer going to be allowed to keep chronic pain suffers as lifetime patients. Because patients now have access to the truths about these critical structures in the head and neck,

Send us your stories!

We're putting together a book to share all the wonderful stories of people getting their lives back. As you're sending your story to the media, send a copy to us as well! Be sure to include a signed letter of consent if you would allow your story, name, and photo in the book and/or in our online materials.

Email your story to us: help@stoptheheadache.com.
Or, mail it to: Chronic Pain Solution Center
5966 Santa Monica Blvd.
Milwaukee, WI 53217

as well as access to the self-exam, they will be able to refer themselves to a qualified dentist, even if their own doctor will not refer them.

CALLING ALL DENTISTS WHO TREAT CHRONIC PAIN, TENSION HEADACHES, AND MIGRAINES

For as much as I have hammered on doctors and dentists who neglect to diagnose and treat this issue, I know an army of qualified dentists that already exists. You who have been treating patients for years—despite the obstacles insurance companies throw in your practice—you are to be commended. I hope you and your patients will join this cause and help lead the charge to save billions more chronic sufferers from a lifetime of pain. Please email us at help@stoptheheadache.com and give us your contact information as well as tell us what skills you can offer to facilitate in this mission.

PATIENTS: If your dentist has treated you well, share your story with us! The more people who rally to this cause, the better. We want to stop the insurance companies from standing in the way of patients getting treatment. To make real change, we need dentists to unite on your behalf.

STOPPING THE EPIDEMIC

I have been successfully relieving patients of chronic pain, tension headaches and migraines for almost forty years. The number of patients we're not able to help significantly without drugs is almost too small to mention. In my entire career, in this legalistic society I've had one lawsuit that I won on all counts. My clinic, The Chronic Pain Solution Center has an excellent rating with the Better Business Bureau. If we were not getting excellent results in a practice where 90 percent of my treatment time is devoted to chronic pain relief, I would have had many suits and complaints. Instead, I have a long list of happy patients who have been freed from the prison of pain. Why? Because I offer a surgery-free, drug-free, long-term solution to chronic suffering.

Give yourself hope! View the book trailer and documentary at stoptheheadache.com. Hear stories from people who have been cured from migraines and chronic pain.

Unfortunately, I also know of many sad patients who were never able to go ahead with treatment. Their insurance companies denied treatment, and these suffering patients couldn't afford to go forward on their own. Most of these patients are so financially tapped out from years of medical bills by the time they find us they're unable to go forward with the treatment.

Now comes the exciting part. We have the opportunity to change the world of medicine, dentistry, and insurance forever. We have the opportunity to stop this epidemic and free not only million and possibly billions of patients today, but billions more in the generations to come from these prisons of pain. This pandemic is so huge, I'm certain that everyone reading this book personally knows at least two to four people who suffer from many of these symptoms. These aren't just numbers. These are real people, moms, dads, children, and grandparents, who can get their lives back.

By making our voices heard, we can force these Goliaths of medicine, dentistry, the insurance industry, the pharmaceutical industry and Congress to release the stranglehold they have on suffering patients. To be effective in this mission, we need massive numbers of involved people, their political and media contacts, and the viral nature of social media to spread like a firestorm across the Internet to overwhelm these Goliaths with unprecedented public opinion. To be sure, once the world realizes how long this practice of pain for profit has been perpetrated, public opinion should be overwhelmingly against the status quo of bottom-line medicine that allows doctors to ignore the issue and allows such suffering to continue.

You must be aware that a mega-profit machine like this is not going to be halted on its own volition. Critics will call me a liar and try to negate the truths in this book. The problem for them is my patients and thousands like them offer walking, talking proof of these truths. That's why we need your help. I have finally come to a point in my life where I cannot allow this injustice to continue. I would have folded against the odds twenty-five years ago if this were just a job, but it isn't. I believe it is my calling to make this treatment, this cure, known. It won't be easy. But giving people back their lives and restoring them to their families healthy and whole is worth the time, effort, and risk. These giants can squelch a handful of people, but when we raise our voices together, the world will have no choice but to listen. Try to imagine the sound of billions of voices making their presence known!

If you're suffering, seek treatment and then make your life-freeing experience known. Watch the video at StopTheHeadache.com to see how others are making their voices heard. Help spread the message of this book. Be courageous! If we do nothing, billions more will suffer. But if we work together, we can stop this epidemic of pain.

The Mission:

- **To open eyes that are blind** (help the world see this problem, and empower people to examine themselves for this problem if their doctors won't).
- **To free captives from prison, and to release from the dungeon those who sit in darkness** (free the billions who suffer in prisons of pain).
  —adapted from Isaiah 42:7

**"Loyalty to a petrified opinion
never broke a chain
or freed a human soul."**
—Mark Twain

ACKNOWLEDGEMENTS

Thank you to all my mentors. I feel truly blessed to have been able to help so many people to get back their lives over the past thirty-eight years. I can only imagine what you went through in the early days of this treatment.

My mentors were teaching about TMJoints and their relationship to migraines and chronic pain when I was still a young pup in dentistry. I owe my passion for treating chronic pain patients to the first man I heard speak at a table clinic in 1974 (I'm sorry to say I don't even know his name), as well as to Dr. Harold Gelb, Dr. Schroeder, Dr. George Eversahl, Dr. Peter Neff, Dr. Bruce Bartos, Dr. James Lampman, Dr. Nathan Shore, Dr. Jerry Murphy, Dr. Jack Hayden, Dr. Brendon Stack, Dr. William Holt, and many, many others. I'd like to think each generation will take it to another level. I hope, after all your frustrations over the years, you're happy about this courageous, but not politically correct or traditional book and effort to finally bring this treatment to the forefront of every physical and dental examination.

I'm also appreciative of the work of the American Academy of Craniofacial Pain, *TMD Diary*, and the *Cranio Journal* for remaining stalwart in their resolve to bring this to the profession of dentistry and the world.

A special thanks goes to the developers of the Tekscan bite computer and the people from Bio Research for their state-of-the-art diagnostic computer software. I believe every dentist should have the TekScan computer system in his or her practice.

Dr. Terrance Spahl for being my expert witness in the only lawsuit I've had in thirty-eight years. We won on all counts.

Popp dental supply for being supportive over the lean years.

Additionally I'd like to thank:

My wife, Holly, for her steadfast courage, powerful prayers, and never losing faith in me or questioning whether what I believed was right, even at times when her home was at risk. Alongside every world changing man is a strong woman.

My six talented children without whom the book, the documentary would never have been within my financial or technical capabilities:

My son Robb who realized that the iPhone and iPad would make history and got us all in on the ground floor. He was right: They are like having extra brains. I never lost an idea or insight. I had a folder or an app for it. I guess I'm thanking Steve Jobs as well.

My son Toben who is a director in Los Angeles. He directed the entire documentary and presented it to me for Christmas 2012.

My daughter Kailey who is a photographer for Missions International and for artists in Nashville. She was the director of photography on the documentary, and my photographer for speaking engagement photos.

My son Jeremy who is an animation director in Atlanta and he's provided me with numerous illustrations and cover design.

My son Tyler who is a partner in a company called Aloompa that designs apps for the iPhone. He's my own private 24/7 AppleCare tech support. He designed the website, blog, Twitter and Facebook pages, and branded them all for *Stop the Headache*. This book was not written without all the technical support and patience Tyler took to keep me up to date in this computerized world.

Last, but certainly not least, my oldest son Pastor Case whose very powerful prayers and counsel during the hard times enabled the whole family. The power of prayer in a family this size is amazing.

Acknowledgements

Rich Muggli, the owner of Muggli Dental Studios, Milwaukee, WI, worked hand in hand with me on some very technical cases over the last 25 years enabling me to try different things and pioneer techniques that differ at times from standard dentistry. And he has given me many breaks over the years to enable me to think outside the box and keep changing the norm.

Mrs. Posse, my sixth-grade teacher who kept the whole class after school for two months writing sixty sets of multiplication tables. I rarely received less than an A in math and science after that.

Georgia, the best teacher I ever had. She was the college instructor who taught this inner city boy he could still get A's and B's competing against students from the suburbs who already had taken calculus and advanced chemistry in high school. She later became my office manager for 17 years. She believed in what I was doing in the early years when no one believed in me. She witnessed firsthand the life-changing miracles of freeing patients of pain and drugs.

An attorney from my church who gave me free legal advice in two major battles. He helped me with a major attack by an insurance company, and the other in the only lawsuit of my chronic pain career. We won them both, in no small part because of his advice. I would not still be standing, and this book would not be coming out were it not for him.

Dr. Larry Nosse, without whom this book would be coming out years later. Larry has his doctorate in physical therapy and is a retired professor of physical therapy at Marquette University. He has been a supportive patient and friend for 40 years. He went to the library and researched endlessly for articles and studies supporting our truths. Thank you Larry, a thousand times over.

Lisa Sterling, invaluable friend, "girl Friday" and office manager all-in-one five-foot dynamo. She did not walk out on me like many others did when the insurance industry set up roadblock after roadblock and

237

made her job miserable, or when the economy went south in 2008. She filled in the gaps of others and literally ran the entire practice without complaining. Instead, we managed to laugh everyday. Because you hung in there this book is going to change the lives of hundreds of millions of people. Your name will be on the rolls that really count.

Kathy C., a writing specialist and dear friend, who reviewed and corrected many of the early chapters. She complimented and corrected an inner city kid's writing ability and gave me wings to continue.

Nancy, the office manager for the Greater Milwaukee Dental Association, who after reading a compassionate letter I wrote about a patient, said, "That is the kind of dentist I want to go to." She became a patient forty years ago and referred numerous people early on to give my practice a start. She has remained a faithful patient all these years while knowing most of the dentists in the Milwaukee area.

Anita, I can't thank you enough for all your help.

My mother, Mabel Seymour, who not only shared her faith with me, but she taught me the secret of life: daily renewal every morning by reading the wisdom and insights of the Bible.

God has provided me with unbelievable people to fill in the gaps for my shortcomings. Without them and my daily renewal for fifty years, I am not standing alone against these Goliaths, let alone having the courage to write this book that challenges the Goliaths of the medical and pharmaceutical industries. Over these fifty years, wisdom has been revealed to me that has been there since the beginning of man. I believe my enamel hypoplasia and poor background blessed me with this problem so that I could learn about it from the inside out. It has opened a life for me that could free hundreds of millions from the prisons of chronic pain, endless drugs and medical bills. Through daily renewal I was able to turn this hardship into a lifelong blessing.

BIBLIOGRAPHY

1. Gorman, Christine; Parr, Alice (October 7, 2002) "The New Science of Headaches," *TIME* magazine (Vol. 160, No. 15), pp. 76-82.

2. Adler, Jerry; Rogers, Adam. (January 11, 1999) "The new war against migraines" Cover story in *Newsweek*. New York: (Vol. 133, No. 2) pp. 46-52.

3. American Migraine Foundation, (January, 14, 2013) "About Migraine." http://www.americanmigrainefoundation.org/about-migraine

4. Armijo-Olivo, Susan; Silvestre, Rony; Fuentes, Jorge, da Costa; Bruno, R.; Gadotti, Inae C.; Warren, Sharon; Major, Paul W.; Thie, Norman M.R.; Magee, David J. (August 2011) "Electromyographic Activity of the Cervical Flexor Muscles in Patients With Temporomandibular Disorders While Performing the Craniocervical Flexion Test: A Cross-Sectional Study," *Physical Therapy* (Vol. 91, No. 8), pp. 1184-1197.

5. Zafar, H. (2004) "Integrated Jaw and Neck Function in Man: Studies of mandibular and head-neck movements during jaw opening-closing tasks," *Swedish Dental Journal*, 2000; Supplement 143; pp. 1-41.

6. Oatis, Carol A. (2004) *Kinesiology: The Mechanics & Pathomechanics of Human Movement*, Lippincott Williams & Wilkins, Philadelphia, PA.

7. Gelb, Harold, D.M.D. (1977) *Clinical Management of Head, Neck and TMJ Pain and Dysfunction*, Philadelphia, PA: W. B. Saunders Company, p. 74.

8. Ventura, Dr. Joseph (2005) "A New Therapeutic Weapon To Reverse Forward Head Posture—Posture Blocks." http://www.posturepro.com/postureblocks.htm

9. Campbell, Dr. Harry (1894) *Headache and Other Morbid Cephalic Sensations,* Chapter 12, "Disorders of the Teeth," London: H. K. Lewis.

10. Weinberg, B. W. (1948) *The History of Dentistry,* Volume 1. St. Louis: C. V. Mosby, pp. 390.

11. Vesalius, Andres (mid-1500s) identified and named the trigeminal nerve and traced it to teeth. http://vesalius.northwestern.edu/index.html

12. Campbell, J. (1958) "Distribution and Treatment of Pain in Temporomandibular Arthroses, "British Dental Journal, Volume 105, pp 393-402.

13. Shore, Nathan Allen, D.D.S., F.A.C.D., F.I.C.D. (1976) *Temporomandibular Joint Dysfunction and Occlusal Equilibration* (Second Edition), Philadelphia and Toronto: J. B. Lippincott Company. pp. 52-55, 128-129, 132, 147-149, 233-34.

14. Funt, Lawrence A., Stack, Brendon C., Directors of the National Capital Center for Craniofacial Pain (December 1977) "Bar Graph of the Evolution of Craniomandibular Pain Syndrome," contributing author Gelb, Harold, D.M.D. *The Clinical Management of Head, Neck and Jaw Dysfunction,* W. B. Saunders, pp. 535.

15. Angell, Marcia, M.D. (2005) *The Truth About Drug Companies, How They Deceive Us And What To Do About It,* New York: Random House Publishing.

16. Porth, Carole Mattson. (2007) *Essentials of Pathophysiology: Concepts of Altered Health States* (Second Edition), Philadelphia, PA: Lippincott Williams & Wilkins, p. 559.

17. Scrivani, Steven J., D.D.S., D.Med.Sc.; Keith, David A., B.D.S., D.M.D.; Kaban, Leonard B., D.M.D., M.D. (December 18, 2008) "Temporomandibular Disorders" *The New England Journal of Medicine,* pp. 2693-2705.

18. Shimshak, Daniel G., M.B.A., Ph.D.; DeFuria, Maureen C., M.S. (July 1998) "Health Care Utilization by Patients with Temporomandibular Joint Disorders," *The Journal of Craniomandibular Practice* (Vol. 18, No. 3), pp.185-193, p. 189.

19. Campbell, Harry, M.D. F.R.P.C. (October 3, 1914) "Discussion On Headache, It's Causes and Treatment," *The British Medical Journal*, p. 581.

20. Campbell, Harry, M.D. F.R.P.C. (October 3, 1914) "Discussion On Headache, It's Causes and Treatment," *The British Medical Journal*, pp. 758-783.

21. Prentiss, H. J. (1918) "A Preliminary Report Upon the Temporomandibular Articulation in the Human Type," *Dental Cosmos* (Vol. 60), pp. 505-514.

22. Costen, James B., M.D. (March 1934) "A Syndrome of Ear and Sinus Symptoms Dependent Upon Disturbed Function of the Temporomandibular Joint," *St. Louis Ann Otol Rhinol Laryngol* (Vol. 43, No. 1), pp. 1-15. http://www.odontocat.com/costen.htm

23. Simmons III, H. Clifton, D.D.S.; Gibbs, S. Julian, D.D.S., Ph.D. (April 2005) "Anterior Repositioning Appliance Therapy for TMJ Disorders: Specific Symptoms Relieved and Relationship to Disk Status on MRI," *The Journal of Craniomandibular Practice* (Vol. 23, No. 2), pp. 89-99.

24. World Health Organization (October 2012) "Headache Disorders" Fact Sheet No. 277. http://www.who.int/mediacentre/factsheets/fs277/en/

25. Stovner, L.J.; Hagen, K.; Jensen, R.; Katsarava, Z.; Lipton, R.; Scher A.I.; Steiner, T.J.; Zwart, J.A. (2007) "The global burden of headache: a documentation of headache prevalence and disability worldwide," *Cephalalgia* (Vol. 27), pp. 193-210.

26. (Winter 2007) "An Interview With ADA President," *Dental Images,* Marquette University School of Dentistry magazine, pp. 14-15.

27. (October 2009) *Journal of Craniomandibular Practice* (Vol. 20, No. 4) p. 231, pp. 235-239, p. 240. pp. 248-249.

28. (1997) "Treatment for the Correction of Temporomandibular Disorders" Assembly Bill 100 section 4930t.632.895 (11) of the statutes, pp. 728-729.

29. (1997) "Can't exclude dentists from treating headaches and chronic pain" Assembly Bill 100 section 632.87 (4)

30. Lexchin, Joel; Bero, Lisa A.; Djulbegovic, Benjamin; Clark, Otavio (May 29, 2003) Abstract: "Pharmaceutical industry sponsorship and research outcome and quality: systematic review." http://www.bmj.com/content/326/7400/1167

31. Aetna Clinical Policy Bulletin Number: 0028: Temporomandibular Disorders, Policy History Last Review: 03/22/2011 Effective: 08/01/1995, Next Review: 01/13/2012 Policy Notes: Most Aetna HMO plans exclude coverage for treatment of temporomandibular disorders (TMD) and temporomandibular joint (TMJ) dysfunction.

32. Chim, H.; Okada, H.C.; Brown, M.S.; Aleyne, B.; Liu, M.T.; Zweibel, S.; Guyuron, B. Source: Department of Plastic Surgery, Case Western Reserve University, Cleveland, OH. "The auriculotemporal nerve in etiology of migraine headaches: compression points and anatomical variations." http://www.ncbi.nlm.nih.gov/pubmed/22842409

33. Tfelt-Hansen, P.; Steiner, T.J. Abstract: "Over-the-counter triptans for migraine: What are the implications?" Department of Neurology, Danish Headache Centre, University of Copenhagen, Glostrup Hospital, Glostrup, Denmark. http://www.ncbi.nlm.nih.gov/pubmed/17927293

34. Stokes, M.; Becker, W.J.; Lipton, R.B.; Sullivan, S.D.; Wilcox, T.K.; Wells, L.; Manack, A.; Proskorovsky, I.; Gladstone, J.; Buse, D.C.; Varon, S.F.; Goadsby, P.J.; Blumenfeld, A.M. "Cost of health care among patients with chronic and episodic migraine in Canada and the USA: results from the International Burden of Migraine Study." http://www.ncbi.nlm.nih.gov/pubmed/21762134

35. Simmons III, H. Clifton, D.D.S. (January 2012) "A Critical Review of Dr. Charles S. Greene's Article titled 'Managing the Care of Patients with Temporomandibular Disorders: A New Guideline for Care: and a Revision of the American Association for Dental Research's 1996 Policy Statement on Temporomandibular Disorders," *The Journal of Craniomandibular Practice* (Vol. 30, No. 1), pp. 9-24.

36. Bevilaqua-Grossi, D.; Lipton, R.B.; Napchan, U.; Grosberg, B.; Ashina, S.; and Bigal, M.E. (February 2010) "Temporomandibular disorders and cutaneous allodynia are associated in individuals with migraine," *Cephalalgia*. http://cep.sagepub.com/content/30/4/425

37. Shimshak, Daniel, G., M.B.A., Ph.D.; Kent, Ralph L., Sc.D.; DeFuria, Maureen, M.S. (1997) "Medical Claims Profiles of Subjects with Temporomandibular Joint Disorders," *The Journal of Craniomandibular Practice* (Vol. 15, No. 2), pp. 150-158.

38. Demerjian, Garabed Gary; Sims, Anthony Benjamin; Stack, Brendan Curran (January 6, 2011) "Proteomic Signature of Temporomandibular Joint Disorders (TMD): Toward diagnostically predictive biomarkers." http://www.ncbi.nlm.nih.gov/pmc/articles/PMC3043347/

39. Gray, Henry, F.R.S. (1966) *Gray's Anatomy* (28th Edition), Editor Charles Mayo Goss, A.B., M.D., Lea & Febiger: pp. 927-928.

40. Nussbaum, Rhoda, M.D. (Summer 2000) "Studies of Women's Health Care: Selected Results," *The Permanente Journal* (Vol. 4, No. 3), p. 61. http://xnet.kp.org/permanentejournal/sum00pj/studies.html

41. Steinbruegge, Jill M., M.D. (Summer 2000) "Commentary: Women's Health—It's More Than Ob-Gyn," *The Permanente Journal* (Vol. 4, No. 3), p. 60. http://thepermanentejournal.org/files/PDF/Summer2000.pdf

GLOSSARY

Apnea: temporary cessation of breathing during sleep.

Auriculotemporal nerve: a branch of the mandibular branch of the TNS that supplies the TMJoints and is repeatedly compressed and irritated when these joints are dislocated. When the TMJoints are dislocated this branch of the TNS is rubbed against and irritated hundreds of times per day/night.

Botox (botulinum toxin): one of the most deadly toxins known to man. It's used in chemical warfare, and now they inject a version of this toxin into the muscles around the eyes and temples to temporarily paralyze facial muscles for a few months at a time.

Bruxing/bruxism: involuntary or habitual grinding of the teeth, typically during sleep.

Canines: see cuspids

Condyle: a rounded protuberance of the lower jaw that functions against the bone in the fossa at the base of the skull, and 2mm from the brain.

Crepitus: a grating sound caused by friction between the condyle and fossa of the TMJoints when the disc or cartilage that is supposed to separate them is dislocated.

Crossbite: a malocclusion (poor bite) where the lower tooth or several teeth fit together outside of the upper teeth. This is the reverse of normal and instills the desire to clench and grind the teeth leading to muscle spasms, strained joints and numerous pain symptoms. (See photos in self-exam.)

Cuspids: pointed teeth, also called canines or eye-teeth, at the rounded corners of the upper and lower arch. They are the most important teeth in the mouth in the prevention of chronic pain and headaches. When the lower jaw grinds to the left or right they cause the upper and lower twelve-year (or second molars) and all the back teeth to separate and function smoothly rather bump into or interfere with the immovable fixed upper opposing teeth at forces that are hundreds of pounds per square inch in the back of the mouth, capable of triggering headaches for decades.

Dental arch: the curvature of an arch that both the upper and lower teeth make in the mouth.

Dowager's Hump: a forward curvature of the spine resulting in a hump at the base of the neck. The medical profession solely blames this on osteoporosis. In *many* cases though, people with a dowager hump have a very small or retruded chin meaning their teeth align in a class 2 retruded bite (the lower jaw is too far back).

Electromyography (EMG): a test to record and evaluate the electrical activity in skeletal muscles.

Equilibration: spot grinding and balancing the height of the teeth and the immediacy of the guidance systems within the bite down to thousandths of a millimeter. In our office this is done using the Tekscan bite computer.

Eustachian: the canal from the pharynx to the middle ear cavity, permitting equalized pressure on each side of the eardrum. When TMJoints are dislocated they are often swollen and causing stuffy ears, tinnitus, and hearing loss.

Fibromyalgia: a disorder characterized by muscular and skeletal pain, fatigue and tenderness. Eighty percent of fibromyalgia patients have TMJ history.

"Follow the money": a money trail leading to who most benefits.

Ganglions (ganglia): a structure containing nerve cell bodies, forming a swelling on a nerve fiber that functions as an amplifier to the impulses. In this case the pain impulses.

Glenoid Fossa: a depression in the floor of the skull within which the condyle of the mandible functions.

Gnathological treatment: a special part of dentistry in which the dentist measures the interactions of the jaw to discover the cause of such health problems as facial pain, TMJ and headaches. You could call it dental structural engineering.

Incisor: the four front lower and upper narrow-edged teeth at the front of the mouth used for cutting or biting off things.

Lacrymal gland: the gland that causes dry eyes or excessive tearing controlled by the TNS.

Lingual: pertaining to the tongue or side of the teeth toward the tongue.

Mandible: lower jaw or jawbone.

Malocclusion: an imperfect bite that displaces and poorly positions the teeth, jaws, TMJoints and muscles at the moment of impact between the upper and lower arches of teeth, and generally results in poor guidance systems and increased possibilities for chronic pain.

Masseter muscle: The strongest muscle in the body used for chewing food and clenching. It is capable of generating forces of hundreds of pounds of pressure per square inch in the back of the mouth.

Ménières disease: disorder of the inner ear characterized by episodes of vertigo, tinnitus and hearing loss. Rarely examined by the medical community, it presents the worst symptom you can get from dislocated TMJoints and irritated TNS.

Neuralgia: intense, intermittent pain along the course of a nerve.

Occipital: the back of the head.

Opthalmic: related to the eye and its diseases. It is also one of the three major branches of the TNS that is responsible for the light sensitivity and intense "ice pick" type pain that migraine patients describe in their eyes.

Orthodontics: a branch of dentistry that deals with correcting malocclusions of the bite with the use of braces.

Overbite: When teeth are closed together the upper teeth deeply overlap or cover half or more of the lower front teeth. (See photos in self-exam.) The upper teeth ideally should cover only about 2mm of the top of the lower teeth.

Overjet: The upper front teeth do not contact the lower front teeth when jaws are closed. (See photos in self-exam.)

Pathologic torque: a twisting force between two poorly aligned teeth affecting the muscles, jaws and joint. It often becomes a clenching and grinding habit.

Prognathic bite: the lower jaw protrudes forward in front of the upper front teeth and jaw.

Proprioceptive: a sensory receptor, found chiefly in muscles, tendons, joints, teeth and the inner ear, that detects the motion or position of the body and body parts, such as the lower jaw, TMJoints and powerful muscles of mastication.

Prosthesis: an artificial device used to replace a missing body part such as a broken down or lost tooth or teeth.

Retruded (opposite of protruded): the lower teeth and jaws line up farther back than they should relative to the alignment of the upper teeth and jaw. Patients with retruded jaws comprise the majority of TMJoint cases and chronic pain.

Sagittal plane: a longitudinal plane that divides a body into right and left sections.

Scoliosis: an abnormal lateral curvature of the spine.

Shimstock articulating strips: a coated, metallic film to test contact points when balancing the bite, as well as dental bridges and crowns that is 1/5000th mm thick.

Sinusitis: inflammation of the sinuses or nasal region.

Splint: a custom fit, removable orthotic that fits over the lower or upper teeth that is used as a diagnostic aid to locate the triplane comfort position (the "Happy Place") of the mandible and both jaw joints. The splint is used to establish that position before making any permanent prosthetic changes to the teeth.

Spur: a bony protuberance or outgrowth often seen on x-rays of the cervical vertebrae of patients who have had the forward and lateral head posture (curved spine) for years.

Sternocleidomastoid muscle: a muscle in the neck that serves to flex and rotate the head.

Tekscan® or T-Scan® computer (TekScan III): a diagnostic bite computer that enables a dentist to measures bite forces, timing and location of these forces or lack of support throughout the mouth. Using computer sensors it is much more accurate than articulating paper (red and blue), and it can display functional movies and timing of guidance systems that can free these patients from the prison of chronic pain.

Temporalis muscle: a large clenching and chewing muscle located precisely in the temple region where many migraine and tension headache patients get the pain. (See photos in self exam.)

Temporomandibular joint (TMJoint): the joint formed by the temporal bone of the skull functioning with the condyle of the mandible. It plays a major role in the assaults on the TNS and the chronic pain symptoms listed in this book.

Tic douloureux (French): trigeminal neuralgia, an acute spasmodic episode of pain along the trigeminal nerve. Severe pain.

Tinnitus: a ringing, buzzing, or whistling sound in the ear caused by an infection, certain drugs, blocked ear canal or head injury. Also caused by dislocated TMJoints and the swelling that accompanies these dislocations that lie 2 millimeters from the ear. As with headaches, no one examines the TMJoints as a cause of tinnitus.

TMJoints: abbreviation for temporomandibular joint.

TN: abbreviation for trigeminal nerve.

TNS: abbreviation for trigeminal nerve system.

Trigeminal nerve system: largest of the 12 cranial nerves. It is also called the chief sensory nerve of the head and face largely because 50 percent of the information going to the brain goes through the TNS. It is involved to some extent in all five senses plus balance, and it supplies almost everything in the mouth: teeth, jaw bones, tongue, TMJoints and the most powerful muscles in the body, the chewing and clenching muscles. It is the major cause of migraines, recurring tension headaches and all the symptoms listed in this book.

Vertigo: a sense of whirling and loss of balance. Feeling of uncertainty and sense of falling or the room spinning around. The worst symptom related to this treatment in that you can't safely drive, take care of the kids or go to work.

Wisdom teeth: the four hindmost molars in humans, appearing about age twenty.

ABOUT THE AUTHOR

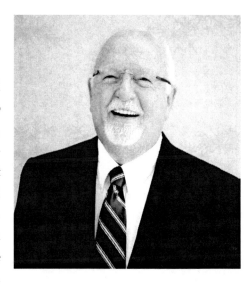

Due to his background of poverty and an inability to afford orthodontics as a child, Dr. Richard T. Seymour experienced the reality and impact of missing and misaligned teeth in a very practical sense. His personal experience with TMJ issues confirmed the need for proper treatment. Studying these problems from the patient's perspective gave him a supreme advantage when he began attending courses related to TMJoint issues. He graduated from Marquette University Dental School in 1970, and spent two years in the dental corps of the United States Air Force.

In practice since 1972, Dr. Seymour has been successfully treating cases of chronic pain for almost 40 years. He has lectured and led discussions on Chronic Pain and TMJ-related neuromuscular disorders and appeared on multiple talk shows regarding a cure for chronic headaches.

He is a member of the Greater Milwaukee Dental Association, the Wisconsin Dental Association, the American Dental Association, and the American Academy of Craniofacial Pain.

His Chronic Pain Solution Center is located in Milwaukee, WI. Learn more at ChronicPainSolutionCenter.com.

GET HELP: STOP THE HEADACHE

If you or a loved one is suffering with chronic headaches, migraines or pain, find a qualified dentist to examine you for TMJ- and TNS-related issues.

If you live in or near Milwaukee, Wisconsin, call or email our office to schedule a consultation.

CHRONIC PAIN SOLUTION CENTER
Phone: 414-961-2484
Email: help@stoptheheadache.com
Website: StopTheHeadache.com

The **AMERICAN ACADEMY OF CRANIOFACIAL PAIN** has a directory of dentists who can examine and treat your TMJ- and TNS-related issues. I encourage you to find a dentist whose practice is significantly (70 percent or higher) devoted to TMD (Temporomandibular Disorders). Visit the patient resources section at **aacfp.org** to access the directory.

12/13-WS

CPSIA information can be obtained at www.ICGtesting.com
Printed in the USA
LVOW06s2134161113

361593LV00024B/1665/P